# 150+ AMAZING USES OF BAKING SODA YOU NEVER KNEW.

(Stunning Uses Of Sodium Bicarbonate In Cleaning, Beauty, Health, Organic, Home, Kitchen, Agriculture, Pesticides etc)

Jane & Richard

# COPYRIGHT 2020

We do not expect part of this book to be reproduced, or transmitted in any form, whether electronics, photocopying or any information storage system without the express permission of the author.

Those who want to review the work are however allowed to quote part of the work in newspapers or magazines.

The book deals with the amazing uses of Baking Soda (Sodium Bicarbonate) including but not limited to uses in the house, for skin and beauty, in the garden and for cars and kids.

They are principally for Home usage but should any reader want to go the business line, such a reader should go by the rules of his country of domain.

Jane Richard.

# DEDICATION.

This book is dedicated to all persons striving to make the world a better place. Those who want to live the word better than they met it.

# ACKNOWLEDGEMENT

We acknowledge the assistance of https://www.freeimages.com/ and Google creatives for the images used in this work.

## SPECIAL NOTICE.

Readers may find that both American and British spellings are used in this book For instance, readers may see color in some places and colour in other places. We crave your indulgence to accept as correct both American and British spellings.

## ACCEPTANCE OF RESPONSIBILITY

We do not lay claim to any perfection, nobody is. Consequently, we accept full responsibility for any deficiency readers might find in this work.

We will cheerfully receive any suggestion to improve on this.

## Contents

**COPYRIGHT 2020**

**DEDICATION.**

**ACKNOWLEDGEMENT**

**SPECIAL NOTICE.**

**ACCEPTANCE OF RESPONSIBILITY**

**1. INTRODUCTION.**

**DESCRIPTION**

**2. HOW TO USE THE BOOK**

**3. HISTORY OF BAKING SODA.**

**4. DIFFERENCE BETWEEN BAKING SODA AND BAKING POWDER**

**5. BAKING SODA (SODIUM BICARBONATE) PROPERTIES.**

**6. CAUTION**

**7. FOR ANIMALS**

   1. Baking Soda Bath For Dogs.

   2. Kennel Beddings And Carpets Need Some Fragrance.

   3. Pet Teeth Cleaning.

   4. Skunk Smell Is Not Good For You.

   5. Wet Bathing For Dogs.

**8. USES FOR BABIES**

   6. Baby Clothes Smell Nice.

7. Baby Flaky Scalp.

8. Remove Diaper Rashes.

9. Baby Bottles Smell Pleasant.

10. Deodorize Diaper Bucket.

11. Pamper Baby's Bum-Bum.

12. Smooth Bath For Baby.

13. Baby's Laundry Too.

## 9. USES IN BEAUTY.

14. A Face & Body Exfoliant.

15. Beautify Your Hands.

16. Clear Your Calluses

17. Black Spots Disappear

18. Dead Skin Cells Are Dead

19. Face Mask, Smooth Face

20. Fights Pimples.

21. Hair In Private Parts?

22. Nail Polish Remnants Suffer

23. Nails Are Whiter

24. No Way For Dandruff

25. Soft Lips kiss Better.

26. Stretch Marks, Go, Go.

27. Sunburn and Sunburn Blisters Cleared.

28. Treats Your Body To A Cheap Fragrance.

29. Under-Eye Treatment.

30. Private Hair Removal 2.

    31.    You Too Deserve Smooth Soles.

## 10. BAKING SODA IN CARS

    32.    Ashtrays To Fragrance

    33.    Car Body Shine Shine

    34.    Car Fragrance For Almost Free

    35.    Car Window Cleaners

    36.    Deodorizes A Smelly Car Boot

    37.    Brighter Headlights And Shining Chrome

    38.    Stop Batteries Terminals Corrosion.

    39.    Stubborn Carpet Stains

    40.    Tape Residue Removal

    41.    Car Leather Treatment

    42.    Sparkling Wheels and Rims

    43.    Seat Belts Are Like New

    44.    Smokers Ashtray And Others.

## 11. BAKING SODA IN FOOD

    45.    Leavening Agent In Bakery.

    46.    Make The Meat Soft And Tender

    47.    Make Your Own Soda Water

    48.    Neutralize Extract Brew

    49.    Softens Beans And Other Hard Cereals

    50.    Stop The Fruits From Going Yellowing

## 12. ............................................................................
## GARDEN.

51. Cabbage Caterpillar Crusher
52. Fire Ants In Trouble
53. Harmful Insect Infestations.
54. Kill Gnats In Compost Heaps
55. Make Garden Furniture Shine
56. Plants Boost
57. Roses will thank you profusely.
58. Treat Tomato Diseases
59. Effective Pesticide.
60. Soil pH Meter.
61. Bouquets Last A Little Longer.

## 13 .HEALTH USES

62. Alkaline water, A Must Have.
63. As Digestive Aid
64. Drop The Fats And Have A Flat Belly.
65. Fight Coughs and Colds
66. Fight Rosacea.
67. Kidney Functions Better
68. Natural Antacid And Acid Reflux
69. Do Nasal Irrigation If You Can.
70. Clear Urinary Tract Infections(UTI)
71. Zaps Ulcer Pain

## 14.
..........................................................................................

## HOME USES.

72. Bathroom Cleaner.
73. Bathroom Curtains Cleaner
74. Bug Repellent
75. Bees Or Insect Stings
76. Clean Brushes And Combs
77. Clean Your Tiles
78. Cleaner In Dishwasher
79. Clear Your Drain
80. Clears Grout Too.
81. Cool Air Freshener For You.
82. Recycling Bin Can Smell Nice/
83. Demolish The Ant Mound.
84. Experience Baking Soda Bath.
85. Fruits Cleaner.
86. Fungicide.
87. Kill Crabgrass And Weeds In Your Lawn.
88. Laundry Bag.
89. Laundry Whitener.
90. Make Everything Sparkle.
91. Old Books Are New.
92. Pests Control
93. Plant And Flower Leaves
94. Insects Repellent
95. Rust Killer
96. Scouring Powder

97. Shine Shine Your Carpet
98. Sparkle Floors
99. Silver Polish
100. Stinky Sneakers
101. Swimming Pool Alkalinity
103. Toilets
104. Toothpaste
105. Towel Cleaner.
106. Wardrobes and Closets
107. Weed Your Sidewalk Weeds
108. Window Cleaners
109. Homemade Toothpaste
110. Computer Cleaning.

**15. WITH KIDS**

111. Baking Soda 'Clay'
112. Bed Wetting Mattresses
113. Clear The Crayon Stains
114. Dolls And Stuffed Animals Get A Bath.
115. Kids Lunch Boxes Smell Nice.

**16. IN THE KITCHEN.**

116. BBQ (Barbecue) Grill
117. Delete Hand Odor
118. Funky-Smelling Dishwasher
119. Garbage Disposals
120. Iron Plate and Coffee Pot Rebirth

121. Plastic Food Storage
122. Pop-Up The Omelette A Bit
123. Make Your Own Fire Extinguisher
124. Multipurpose Kitchen Cleaner
125. Neutralize Fridge Odors
126. Odor-Free Microwaves
127. Scorched Pot Cleaner
128. Sparkle Pots And Pans
129. Stale Smell From Used Containers
131. Thermoses And Flasks Too.
132. Wash The Blender

## 17. PERSONAL HYGIENE

133. Deodorize Your Shoes
134. Fight off Athlete Foot.
135. Make A Deodorant
136. Mouthwash Kills Mouth Odour
137. Sparkling Flatware
138. Splinter Is Out.

## 18. IN SPORTS

139. Cleaner Sports Equipment
140. Electrolyte Booster, Sports Drink

## 19. MORE USES.

141. Hot Water Burn
142. Peel Your Eggs With Ease
143. A Volcano To Thrill The Kids.

144. Reduce Food sour Taste
145. Forget ToothAche
146. Baby Post Eating Fresh-Up
147. Wash Your Private Part {PP}
148. Test For Baby Sex
149. Garden Decorations to Enjoy
150. Treat Cutting Boards
151. Wall Hole got filled up
152. Mobile Air Freshener For You
153. Sports Equipment Remembered
154. Kills Sweet Craving
155. Balloon Blow Blow
156. Gutter Cleaner Is Here
157. Glowing Skin Is Your Right.

**20 CLEVER USES YOU CAN COMMERCIALIZE RIGHT AWAY**

**21. FAQS ON BAKING SODA.**

**22. WRITE A REVIEW.**

**23. .OTHER BOOKS BY THE AUTHOR.**

**20 ABOUT THE AUTHOR.**

# 1.INTRODUCTION.

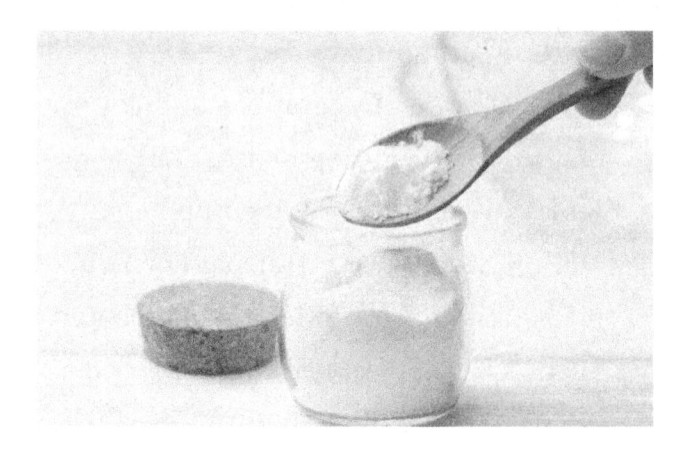

As an SME expert and alternative therapy enthusiast, whenever I come across something, I always think about what ways can this thing be useful as an SME.

You know, to a carpenter, everything looks like a hammer.

And believe me, this has been of tremendous help.

Let me tell you an example.

I bought a local substance from the market for my domestic use one day but for one reason or the other; I deferred the use.

One day, I noticed that rats have ravaged this material where I kept it even as I thought I wrapped it properly.

Then I thought, If rats could go to such an extent to eat this stuff, they would go any length to eat it even if poisoned.

That was the beginning of the well known Last Supper rat poison in the market.

I must confess that I had known about Sodium Bicarbonate, (Baking Soda) since my secondary school days and got to know about it the more in higher institutions as a science student but never knew it could have many industrial uses.

Who would think it could be more useful than its mother sodium carbonate?.

I am not sure God has made any chemical with such diverse uses as Baking Soda. It's a magic powder.

Growing up, I started stumbling on its vast uses domestically and industrially. One day, the SME thing in me asked if all these uses could not be commercialized to make money?

Why not? If you could mix Baking Soda and lime to get something useful in the house, why can't such be commercialized?

I had known all along that what the big companies do is to mix up these common things to put holes in our pocket? It is more of packaging than the material inside.

And as you will find out later, that is what most of them do. That is a fragrance made from ordinary ethanol and a fragrance goes for $6 because of the exotic bottle and box.

If you activate this book, you will not spend your money on many proprietary products as you will make them yourself.

To put these down, I did some research which made me realize that I was just scratching the surface of the uses of baking soda.

There and then I dropped my SME Cap for a while and put on my Chemistry cap.

The result coupled with my experience as a chemist, lecturer, and management consultant is this book "150+ Amazing Uses Of Baking Soda You Never Knew.

If this is all you have and you take action by putting it to use, there is no excuse for you to be poor.

The greatest attribute of this product is its cheapness. It is damn cheap, about N200 per Kg. Coupled with this is that it combines effectiveness with non-toxicity.

If a toddler or pet swallows a pinch, nothing will happen.

One more thing in this book, we go straight to the point, cutting out the frills.

You don't need them.

Good luck.

Jane Richard

# DESCRIPTION

**How would you feel to make use of a very cheap substance in over** 150 ways in your home and environment, saving yourself a lot of money and possibly make some money?

Welcome to the world of Baking Soda (Sodium Bicarbonate) the silky whitish magic powder that is very effective in its many uses, yet non-toxic. And so, so cheap.

A must-have in every household. And with a copy of 150+ Amazing Uses Of Baking Soda You Never Knew, in your hands, you are home and dry.

It is doubtful if God created any substance with more diverse you than Baking Soda, besides water.

Unfortunately, as useful and cheap as Baking Soda is, many people are ignorant of its uses. But not you anymore.

Your book will take you through the exciting journey of Baking Soda uses.

You will discover its incredible uses in Health, Personal Hygiene, beauty, and cleaning that we all need to know.

It will take though its uses, in the house, in the kitchen, in the garden, for your car, for your health and beauty not forgetting your kids and pets. And many more.

If you are the enterprising type, you might even try to convert some uses to money.

The man cleaning your car headlight for money uses Baking Soda.

That and many other applications in the book could be used to make money.

Ok. You are not interested in making money with Baking Soda, what of the money-saving uses?

You use Baking soda to achieve jaw-dropping results compared to the expensive proprietary products you buy outside.

Definitely you would want to save money, who doesn't, anyway?

If, for instance, you make your own toothpaste, skin exfoliator, body fragrance, and deodorizer, you would have saved yourself some dollars.

And trust me, there are more amazing things you can make with 150+ Amazing Uses Of Baking Soda You Never Knew,

Since I became an apostle of this powder, my house is cleaner with a constant pleasant odor.

Not in my house would you find a crawling insect, whether day or night. My car shines all the time and my car headlights stay bright any day.

Oh, my dog, Kim, loves the weekly dry Baking Soda bath which gives her bright shining furs.

With this book, you will have a fresh smelling and sparkle kitchen with Baking soda versatility in the kitchen.

The moment you use Baking Soda, you get positive comments.

See a few of the recipes you get in 150+ Amazing Uses Of Baking Soda You Never Knew,

- Wet Bathing For Dogs
- A Face & Body Exfoliant
- No Way For Dandruff
- Nails Are Whiter
- Stretch Marks, Go, Go
- Car Fragrance For Almost Free
- Make The Meat Soft And Tender
- Soil pH Meter
- Alkaline water, A Must Have.
- Drop The Fats And Have A Flat Belly

Trust me, with 150+ Amazing Uses Of Baking Soda You Never Knew, all things are new. Domestic chores are easier and better.

Your environment is safer and you live a chemical-free life as baking Soda is natural.

All these cheaply because Baking Soda is damn cheap.

The only regret you would have is, why did I not know about Baking Soda and 150+ Amazing Uses Of Baking Soda You Never Knew, before now.

## 2. HOW TO USE THE BOOK

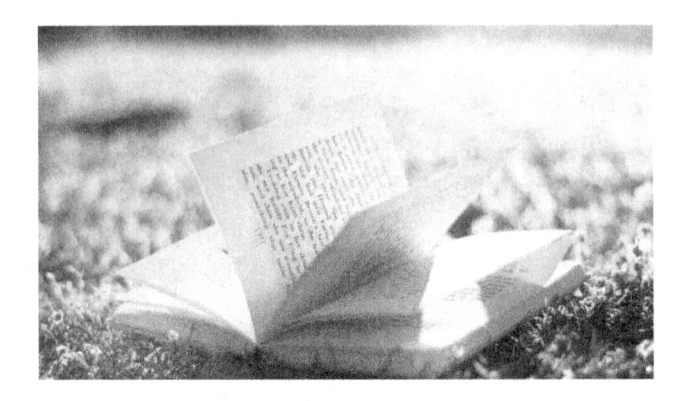

Your book **150+ Amazing Uses Of Baking Soda You Never Knew** is not an academic book. I write it in such a way as to educate and entertain.

Therefore, my advice to you is to read from the beginning to the end in a relaxed mood, if you like.

There are reasons for this. First, you have a general feel of the book.

Second, you may discover that many ideas may be novel to you as I expect but which may interest you and which you may see in a more unique light than I have seen it

Having done that, you may now use the contents to reach the different uses as they interest you.

As you read, make marks of those you admire. The book is like a dictionary which you will need to consult regularly.

You may have hitches, and these are not unusual. When such happens, ask questions and I am here for you.

Call me or send an email.

Heavenly blessings.

Jane Richard.

# 3. HISTORY OF BAKING SODA.

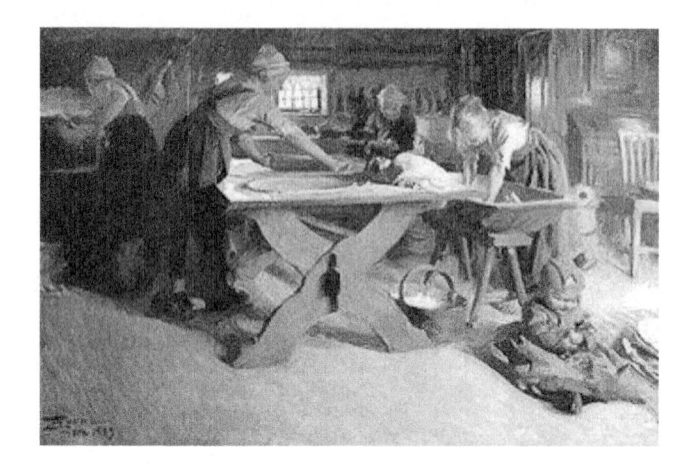

Baking soda comes from two soil minerals called Nahcolite and Trona which are refined into calciumcarbonate which is then turned into Sodium bicarbonate a.k.a Baking Soda.

Around 1791, Nicolas Labnac, a French Chemist produced Sodium carbonate.

In 1846, two brothers-in-law, Dr. Austin Church and John Dwight, established the first Baking Soda factory in the USA and collaborated to distribute it.

We credit the rise of Baking soda to one big brand- Arm & Hammer

To show the people the usefulness of Baking Soda and to popularise it, Arm & Hammer began a marketing campaign in 1860.

They distributed food recipes some of which originated from the family comprising bread, cookies, cakes, puddings recipe.

To spread the popularity, bicarbonate of soda was publicized in the 1920 edition of women's magazine.From then people developed the habit of keeping a box of Baking soda in their homes.

# 4. DIFFERENCE BETWEEN BAKING SODA AND BAKING POWDER

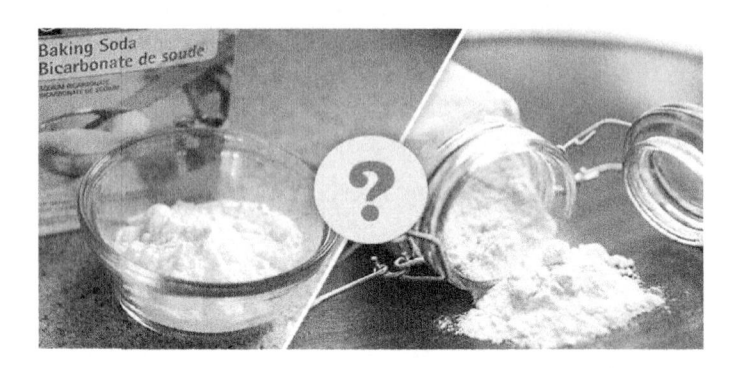

There is a difference between these two chemicals, Baking Soda and Baking Powder.

Unfortunately, many have mistaken one for the other, getting unexpected results.

**So what is the difference?**

Baking Soda, ($NaHCO_3$) also called Soda Ash or Soda Crystals, is just one substance, sodium bicarbonate. Sodium bicarbonate is a base and like all bases, it reacts with acids to form gas and salt.

With Sodium Bicarbonate, the gas it produces is carbon dioxide ($CO_2$).

This is the gas you notice when it is mixed with vinegar.

This quick action gives bakers an enormous problem.

They want even action spread overtime to get their wares done but Baking Soda reaction is effervescent which doesn't go well with baking.

Baking powder solves this problem because it has different ingredients which make it act evenly throughout the baking period.

Some experts say it is "double acting".

All baking powder contains Baking Soda, but they also contain some other chemicals to make baking powder behave the way it does.

These other chemicals (acids) are Monocalcium Phosphate and either Sodium Acid Pyrophosphate or Sodium Aluminium Sulphate.

The earlier acid doesn't react with the sodium bicarbonate while it's dry but will react as soon as the dough is wet while either of the other two will not react until the dough is wet and hot.

Put differently, Sodium Aluminum Sulphate or Sodium Acid Pyrophosphate will not react with Baking Soda until the dough or batter is wet and in the oven.

The result is that the batter or dough rises for a longer time, making lots of bubbles in the process for a better bake.

So baking powder is Baking Soda and some other chemicals.

In some products, Baking Soda may work in place of baking soda but not in health or beauty matters.

Baking soda is a component of baking soda as they manufacture baking Powder from Baking Soda.

Baking soda is a natural product which is the reason baking powder expires in a matter of months while Baking Soda lasts for life.

So be sure of what you are holding.

# 5. BAKING SODA (SODIUM BICARBONATE) PROPERTIES.

## Physical Properties.

These are characteristics you can observe without changing the identity or composition of a substance.

Baking Soda is a white, crystalline powder that forms lumps occasionally.

It is odorless with a bitter, salty taste.

Solid white at room temperature.

Highly soluble in water, but evaporation can separate the two.

## Chemical Properties.

These are properties when a substance changes its chemical composition.

One percent molar solution of Sodium Bicarbonate in water at room temperature has a pH of 8.3. This makes it alkaline and hence the bitter taste.

When heated to above 50 degrees Celsius, Baking soda decomposes to carbon dioxide ($CO_2$) and water ($H_2O$) with traces of Sodium Carbonate.

# 6. CAUTION

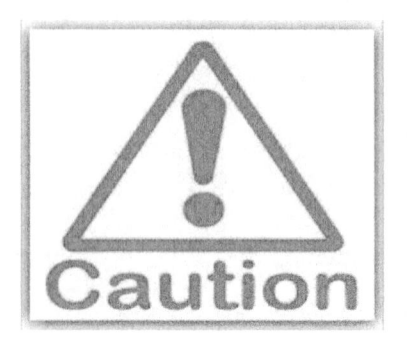

We consider using Baking soda on the body as safe but when you ingest Baking Soda, be very careful.

Too much Baking soda in the system, as we explained elsewhere, can alter the body chemistry and cause hassles.

Baking soda is high in sodium — 1,259 milligrams in one teaspoon — so high doses are not safe.

Too much baking soda can increase potassium excretion, which could lead to potassium deficiency in the body.

And this is a metal needed for bones and other uses.

People with underlying medical problems such as liver disease, high blood pressure, and kidney disease should not take in baking soda.

And if you are breastfeeding or pregnant, avoid taking it.

If you are on prescription drugs, speak to your doctor before you ingest anything with baking soda.

If you are on a medical treatment using baking soda for two weeks with no improvement. Stop use and consult your doctor.

## AVOID:

- Taking Baking Soda within two hours of taking other medications.
- Taking a solution containing Baking Soda that is not dissolved.
- Taking over 5 teaspoons of baking soda in a day
- Taking over 1.5 teaspoons a day if you are over 60 years old
- Taking baking soda solution too quickly
- Taking baking soda when you are filled up to avoid gastronomic disorder.

# 7. FOR ANIMALS

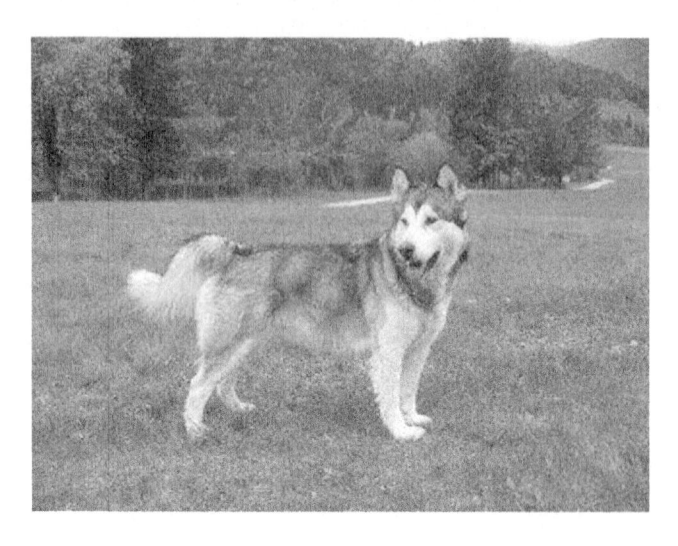

### 1. Baking Soda Bath For Dogs.

You are a dog owner? You can give your dog a dry shampoo bath using our friend Baking Soda instead of spending money at the vet.

Remove loose hairs by brushing the coat.

Wipe his paws, and around his face gently with a warm, damp cloth.

Now sprinkle Baking Soda on the coat but make sure you avoid the face, eyes, and nostrils.

Let the powder stay on for minutes before you use a hand towel to remove the excess powder.

Your dog comes out shining without odor.

I know because I do it for my Rott every Saturday

## 2. Kennel Beddings And Carpets Need Some Fragrance.

If you have a battery of kennels with many dogs, you cannot run away from smells.

Not to worry, Baking Soda is there for you.

Liberally, sprinkle baking soda on all the surfaces you want to be treated. Leave for about 30 minutes and longer, if necessary, then vacuum thoroughly.

You can also use Baking soda to keep the kitty litter box fresh in between changes.

All you need do is add a little Baking Soda to the base and then add the litter later.

## 3. Pet Teeth Cleaning.

You have read how to use baking soda for your teeth and mouth.

It works for your pet teeth too.
See Personal hygiene


## 4. Skunk Smell Is Not Good For You.

If your dog has what we call Skunk smell, you may need additives to Baking soda to fight it.

**This is the recipe.**
- ✓   1 litre of hydrogen peroxide
- ✓   ¼ cup of baking soda.
- ✓   1 teaspoon of grease eating detergent

Mix thoroughly and use to bathe the dog, avoiding the nose and eyes. With a towel, you can gently clean the face after the body bath.

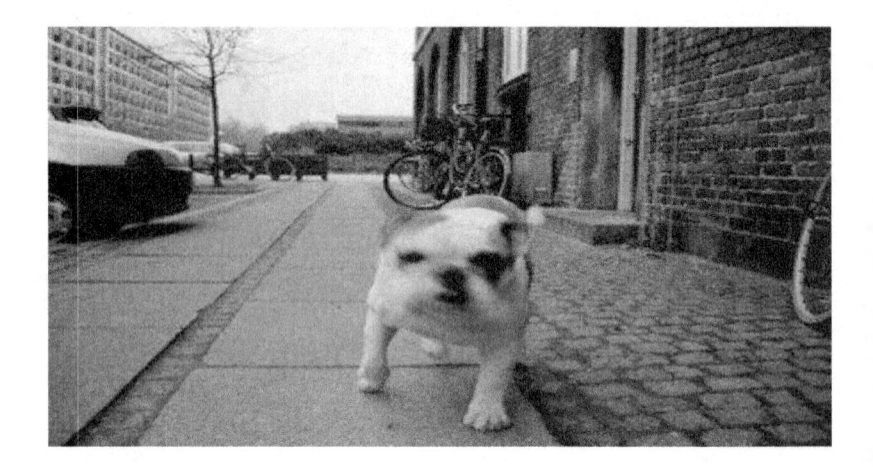

The smell may not go completely at first but will reduce significantly. Continuation for 2 weeks should get the smell off.

The solution can also wash the bedding and clothing that may have been affected.

It can also whiten your laundry.

### 5. Wet Bathing For Dogs.
You know about a dry bath for dogs that make their fur shine.

This is a wet bath for your dog, which you do now and then unless she rolls in dirt or faeces.

- ✓ 3 Tablespoons Baking Soda
- ✓ 1 Litre Of Warm Water.

Wash your dog with the solution, allowing the solution some minutes to eat up the odor.

Wash with clean water severally to be sure the solution is no more on her skin to forestall itching.

Your dog is clean and okay.

# 8. USES FOR BABIES

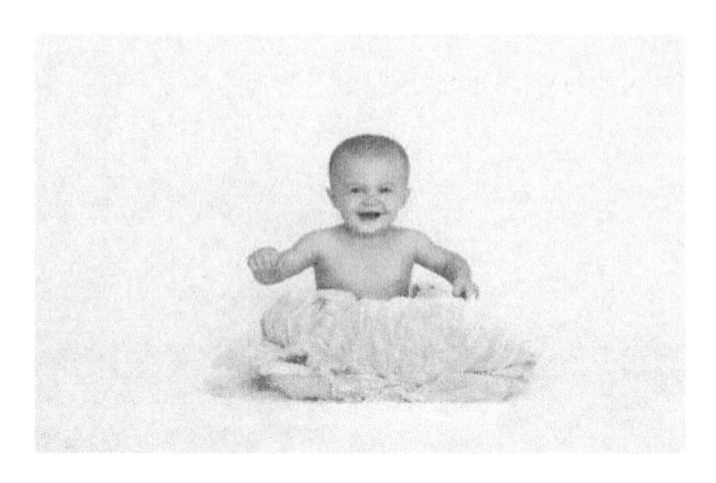

### 6. Baby Clothes Smell Nice.
Some commercial detergents may be too harsh on the baby.

A superb way to remove odor from the baby's clothes is to add Baking Soda to the baby's liquid laundry.

Half a cup of baking soda to the laundry water and detergent will ensure the stains are gone while retaining a fresh odor.

It helps if you add some Baking Soda to the rinse cycle.


### 7. Baby Flaky Scalp.
Baby flaky scalp will go on its own with time with no treatment. But if you are one who cannot stand it and wants it off quickly, this is a Baking Soda recipe to help.

Make a paste of Baking Soda and water in your palm.

Rub gently on the affected area, avoiding the baby's eyes. Wipe off with a damp towel making sure you do not use soap or shampoo.

If the baby's head is red, stop using and replace it with baby oil. The soda may be too harsh for the baby.

### 8. Remove Diaper Rashes.

The red rashes on the bum of babies are diaper rashes. Fight it by using a solution of baking Soda and warm water on the bottom areas.

Baking soda soothes and neutralizes the urine acid.
You can alkaline the baby bath water with 1/2 cup of baking soda.

Don't sprinkle baking soda directly on the baby's skin.

### 9. Baby Bottles Smell Pleasant.

You will need to remove funk from baby's feeding bottles, nipples and all.

Soak overnight in a solution of 4tablespoons of Baking Soda in 1 liter of warm water.

In the morning, wash with hot water and soap. Continue feeding your baby with them.

### 10. Deodorize Diaper Bucket.

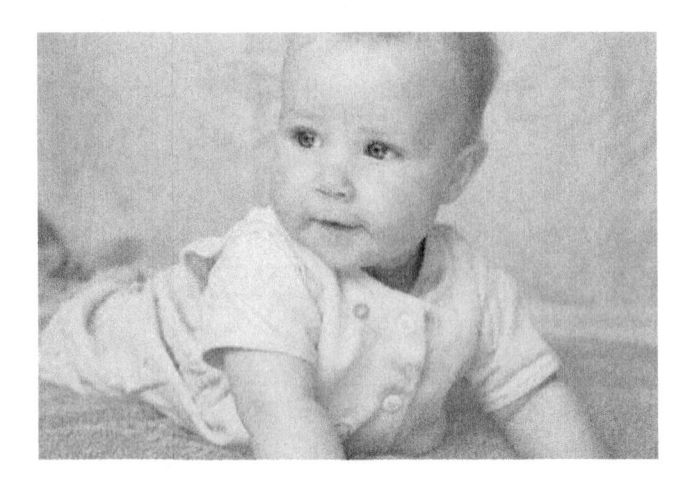

For either cloth or disposable diapers you will do well to sprinkle baking soda into the diapers bucket. It gives you a nice small until you are ready to dispose of the diapers.

As said elsewhere, the diapers will thank you for some Baking soda in their laundry water.

### 11. Pamper Baby's Bum-Bum.

Junior had wet his diapers with the later smelling of Urea.

Not only that, but the urea has also made his bum red. Not to worry, sprinkle Baking soda into the diapers to prevent the rash and the smell.

### 12. Smooth Bath For Baby.

You put Baking soda in your bath water, babies, and kids don't mind it too.

This works for grownups and babies alike. Just a few tablespoons in baby's bathwater to fight diaper rash.

13. Baby's Laundry Too.
Add 1/2 cup of baking soda to a load of laundry. Result-fresh smelling and softer clothes just as adults clothes.

## 9. USES IN BEAUTY.

### 14. A Face & Body Exfoliant.

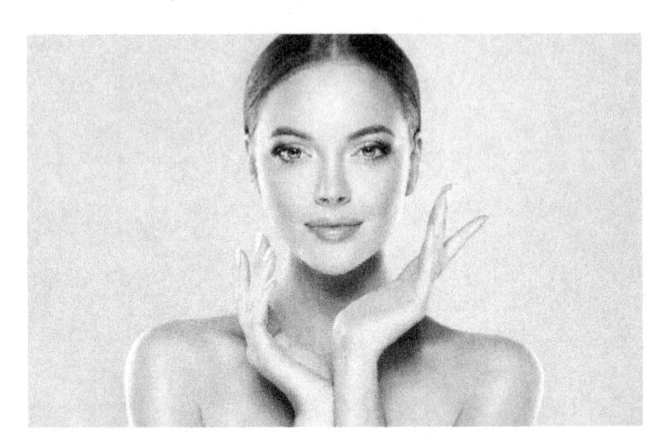

As baking soda does great in cleaning other things, it can also be made to a gentle but effective exfoliant.

In the bath, make a paste of water and Baking Soda in your palm.

Now rub into your skin. It will sting if it gets into your eyes, but flushing with water will take care of that. But soap does that too, and we don't complain.

Leave for a couple of minutes, then wash off with water. You may limit it to your face if you cannot apply to the entire body.

This exfoliant is very effective, so start with one treatment a week and increase its frequency as needed.

### 15. Beautify Your Hands.

Baking soda has an abrasive property which when combined with jelly will make your palm smooth.

It will exfoliate your hand removing the dead cell to give you a smooth palm to the admiration of others.

You have just finished working in the garden, pour a bit of the magic stuff in your hand, add water and scrub.

If you want to scale it up, add little drops of olive oil, petroleum jelly, baby oil or mineral oil and scrub the hands.

Rinse thoroughly with warm water.

Apply a moisturizer because with time the skin will feel dry.

### 16. Clear Your Calluses

Calluses are the hardened area of feet, toes, fingers, and palms caused by frequent frictions.

Although they may not cause issues, pressure on them may be painful.

Soaking your callus-ridden area in a baking soda solution will soften the area where after you can remove the scales and dead cells.

### 17. Black Spots Disappear

If you have black spots on your face, it reduces self-esteem.

You feel inferior if there are black spots on your face. Baking soda can come to your rescue to remove these blemishes and spots.

Baking soda has a bleaching property which may be harsh on the skin but when mixed with another natural bleaching agent-Lemon, it will do the job.

**Recipe: Mix**
- ✓ 1 tablespoon of Baking soda
- ✓ 4 tablespoons of squeezed lemon juice

Mix to get a thick paste
Clean your face and now apply the paste on the blemishes and other parts of the face. Leave for about 5 minutes and then wash with warm water, and later with cold water.

Dry up and add a moisturizer.

Best applied in the night as exposure of lemon to the sun may darken the skin

Apply once or twice a week and experience visible changes.

## 18. Dead Skin Cells Are Dead

Often, dirt, pollution, and grime settle on our faces and they don't come off easily with an ordinary bath or ordinary face wash.

To remove these particles, we need a natural cleanser.

Here again, the exfoliating property of Baking Soda comes to use to remove the dead skin cells and these impurities.

**Recipe.**
- 1 tablespoon of Baking soda
- ½ tablespoon water
- Not too much water, we need a thick paste.
- Wash your face and then apply this paste in circular motions, making sure you don't get it into the eyes.
- Leave for a couple of minutes.
- Useful for oily faces, not dry faces
- Wash off with water and pat dry.
- Apply a moisturizer
- Apply once a week to get a fresh-looking skin.

### 19. Face Mask, Smooth Face

You have seen them making expensive face masks to make their faces beautiful. You too can do it with a cheap recipe getting the same if not better result.

- ✓ ½ teaspoon baking soda
- ✓ ½ teaspoon lemon juice
- ✓ 1 tablespoon honey.

Mix thoroughly and gently apply on the face, allow to sink for 15 minutes and then rinse with water. Apply gently, not scrub.
See smooth face.

### 20. Fights Pimples.

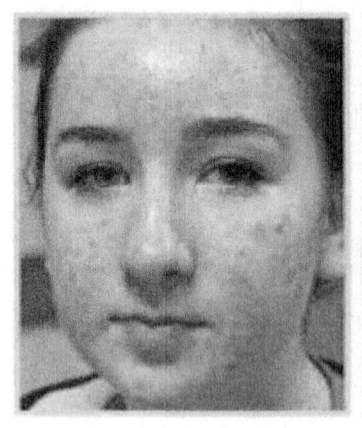

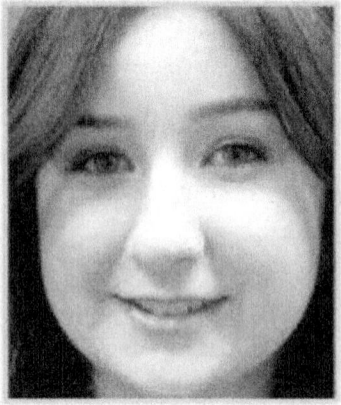

Baking Soda has an exfoliating property which makes it handy in preparation of skincare products. This is the property we are exploiting here.

It dries the pimples and its bactericidal and antifungal property prevents further skin break.

**Recipe.**
- 1 tablespoon of Baking soda
- 1 tablespoon of water.

Mix to a paste.

**Application.** Wash your face properly and apply the paste on pimple or acne.

Leave for 3 minutes, then wash with lukewarm water.

You can also apply an ice cube and if it dries your skin apply a moisturizer.

Use this once or twice a week and watch the acne reduce.

## 21. Hair In Private Parts?

When we have hair in our private parts and armpits, we settle for shaving blades or shaving cream and powders which cost some dough.

You can use cheap Baking Soda to remove these hairs from the private parts.

Natural and very safe. No side effects.
Mix a tablespoon of baking soda with 200 cm3 of water.

**Preparation:**
- ✓ Boil the water
- ✓ Turn the heat off
- ✓ Add baking soda.
- ✓ Mix thoroughly.

**Use:**
- ◆ Apply this solution to the areas with hair before bed in the night.
- ◆ Wash in the morning.
- ◆ Repeat this three times and you will see the hairs off.

## 22. Nail Polish Remnants Suffer

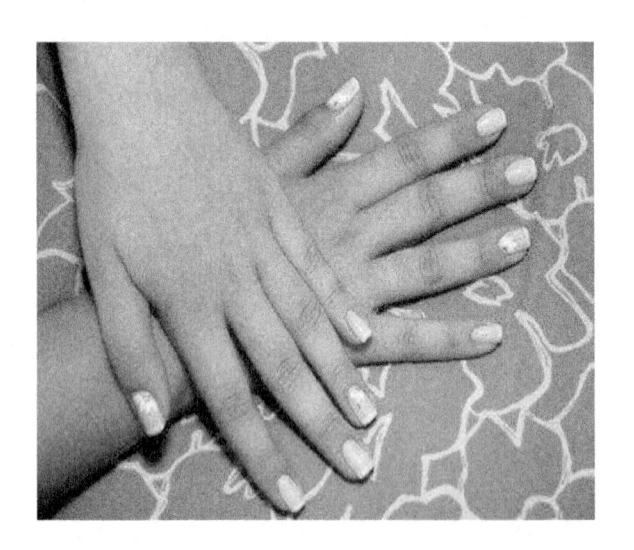

Allow to remain for 10 minutes and wash off.
The result is amazing.

### 23. Nails Are Whiter

You want neater whiter nails. That should not bother you as you have your Baking Soda.

Soak nails for 10 minutes in 4tablespoons of baking Soda and 2 tablespoons of hydrogen peroxide and a half cup of hot water.

The result will surprise you.

### 24. No Way For Dandruff

Baking soda is alkaline, and therefore it has grease and fats removing properties.

And we know grease and oil on the scalp contribute to dandruff.

Being a natural antiseptic, Baking Soda also helps to balance the pH level of the scalp.

These and other properties make baking soda a great anti Dandruff.

**Recipe.**
- ✓ Mix 2 tablespoons of baking soda with water until it gets to be a paste.
- ✓ For perfect results, put some drops of olive oil on the scalp.

Now apply the prepared paste and leave for 5 to 12 minutes. Rinse the mixture out thoroughly.

Do this once or twice a week.

Can you sell this to hairdressers?

### 25. Soft Lips kiss Better.

Some foul habits like Smoking and wearing lipstick for a long time may make your lips thick with black color.

Too much exposure to the sun can also aggravate it.

To get the natural color back and lip softness, go call our friend Baking Soda and one of his friends, pure honey. Honey removes impurities and softens as well.

Since you are working on the lips, you need little.
- ✓ ¼ tablespoon each of honey and Baking soda.
- ✓ Mix to a paste, and add on the lips in a circular motion
- ✓ Leave for a couple of minutes. Then wash off. You may apply a lip balm later.
- ✓ Your lip will get exfoliated and dead cells will vamoose.

- ✓ Do this once or twice a week and get a bright soft lip

### 26. Stretch Marks, Go, Go.

You carry a bulging belly for 9 months, after which you drop a bundle of joy that gladdens people around you.

Often, some marks on the body come with this joy. They are stretch marks.

Baking soda and lemon which has a bleaching property will fight these marks.

Remember Baking Soda is a natural exfoliant that removes the dead cells.

Make a paste of baking soda and lemon and apply on the marks and cover with kitchen foil. Wash after 15 minutes.

First, try on a small portion for a few minutes, if it neither hurts nor itch, you can then apply on the whole.

The recipe has proved effective in removing stretch marks. Can somebody Package this and sell?

### 27. Sunburn and Sunburn Blisters Cleared.

In summer, you need a pack of Baking Soda. Because it is alkaline, it has a soothing smell on skins burned by the sun. It also relieves itching and other burning sensations.

Because of its antiseptic and drying properties, it helps with sunburn blisters.

**Mix**
- ✓ 1 to 2 tablespoons of Baking Soda

- ✓ 1 cup of cold water.

Soak a hand towel in this solution, wring the water out, and now use the damp towel to compress the affected area.

Do this 3ce until you are okay.

**Alternatively,**
½ cup of baking soda to a bathtub filled with water.
Dissolve the powder properly, stir properly.
Soak your body in this solution for 15 minutes or thereabout.
Pat dry your body and allow air to complete the drying.
Once-daily until it relieves you..

Do this once daily for a few days.

### 28. Treats Your Body To A Cheap Fragrance.

Body odor can be embarrassing. Use Baking soda to give your body a pleasant odor cheaply.

- ✓ ⅛ teaspoon of baking soda,
- ✓ 1 tablespoon of water,
- ✓ A few drops of any essential oil.

Rub the mixture on your underarms and areas of your body where you sweat profusely. You have gotten regular body fragrance.

**Alternatively,**

- ✓ Mix 50/50 baking soda and cornstarch.
- ✓ Dust the mixture on your underarms and areas of your body where you sweat profusely.
- ✓

29. Under-Eye Treatment.

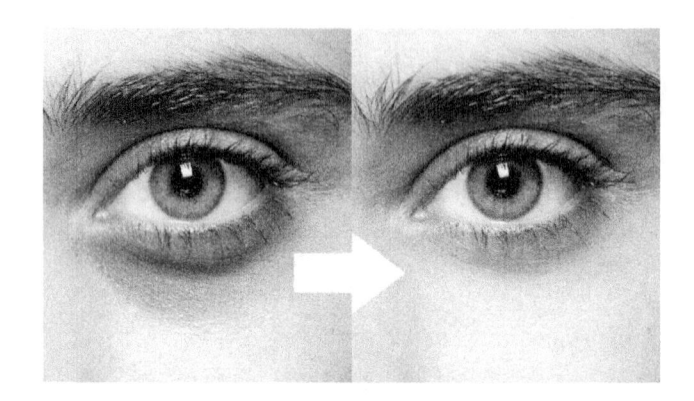

Get rid of the black circles under the eyes.
- ✓ Make a paste of 3 parts baking soda and 1 part water.
- ✓ Apply the paste to the area affected and let it sink for about 7 minutes.
- ✓ Rinse off carefully, making sure it doesn't get into your eye.
- ✓

It won't blind you, but it may hurt.

30. Private Hair Removal 2.

**Recipe**
- ✓ 2 parts baking soda with
- ✓ 1 part turmeric
- ✓ a few teaspoons of water to form a paste.
- ✓

Apply on the unwanted hairs and leave to dry.

Remove the dry paste with a damp towel and wash clean with water to remove the paste and turmeric coloration.

### 31. You Too Deserve Smooth Soles.

You want the sole (under the surface of the feet) to be smooth and clean and fresh?

- ✓ 3 tablespoons of baking soda
- ✓ 1 tablespoon water.

Soak for 15 minutes

Scrub with a sponge, then wash with clean water to prevent itching.

# 10. BAKING SODA IN CARS

### 32. Ashtrays To Fragrance
Most people do not use their ashtrays in the car anymore.

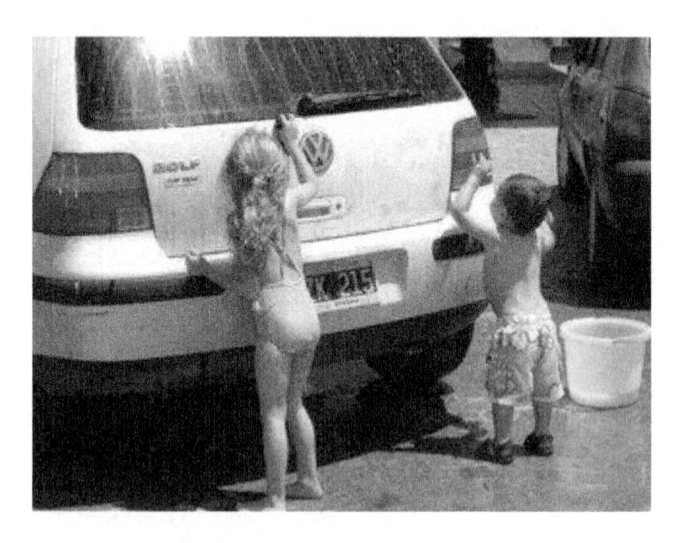

You can use it as a storehouse of fragrance in the car to eliminate odour. You can fill it to ¼ with Baking Soda and enjoy.

No need for expensive fragrance.

See car fragrance.

### 33. Car Body Shine Shine
Our friend Baking soda is abrasive but gentle with it. It's, therefore, the right candidate to remove dirt, tree sap, and

bugs from your car's exterior without doing damage to the finish.
Easy, dip a damp cloth in some baking soda to remove the little annoying blemishes with circular motions. Use water to rinse the area to remove the baking soda.

You can use the same system to clean your headlights and keep them shining and brighter.

OMG, the last time I cleaned my car headlights here, I was charged for it and the guy used a powder. (Baking Soda).

*You can add some baking soda to your car washing water.*

You can make tons of money from this with car owners if you packaged it properly.

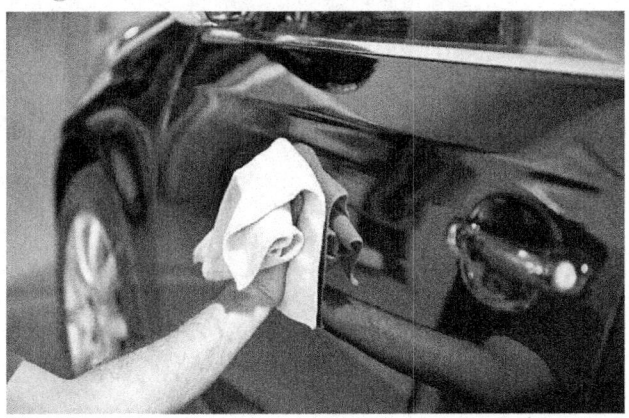

### 34. Car Fragrance For Almost Free

Sprinkle baking soda on your seats, rugs, and carpeting. Leave for a few hours and clean off

It is white and will not stain your seats.

If the odor is coming from a particular corner, put the powder there and forget.

It will suppress the odor

### 35. Car Window Cleaners

One tablespoon of baking soda in 4 cups of warm water will do just nicely.

Mix thoroughly and use to clean car windows and windshields
Windows will remain clean and fight back dirt.

The baking soda will break up road grime and ensure that the windows remain streak-free.

### 36. Deodorizes A Smelly Car Boot

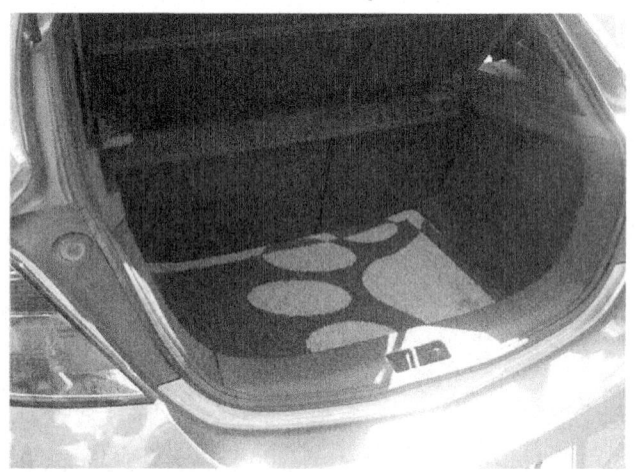

First, wash clean with water and soap, rinse and wipe clean
Wipe with full-strength vinegar and let dry.

Leave the trunk open to dry.

Sprinkle a boxful of baking soda over the area and rub it in with your hands.

50

Leave on for a few days and then vacuum out the baking soda.

Most people do not use their ashtrays in the car anymore.

You can use it as a storehouse of fragrance in the car to eliminate odor. You can fill it to ¼ with Baking Soda and enjoy it.

No need for an expensive fragrance.
See car fragrance.

### 37. Brighter Headlights And Shining Chrome

Elsewhere here I wrote about paying 2000N to make my headlight brighter. I agree they cleaned both the inside and the outside using their powder (Baking soda)

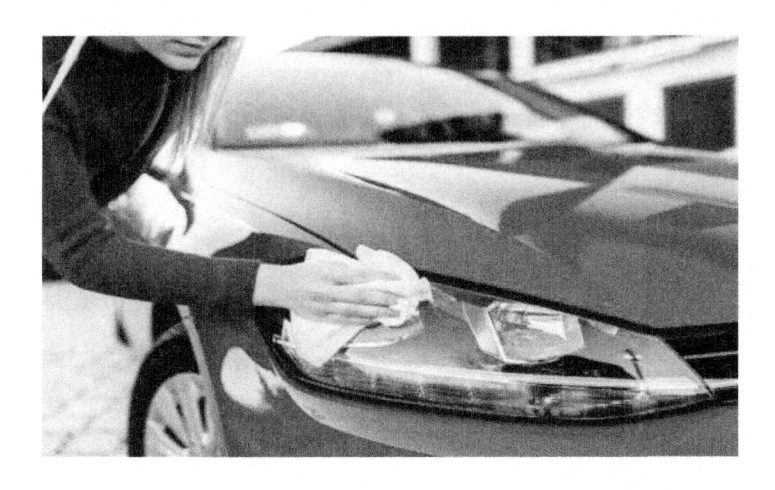

You can do this yourself if you can remove the headlight. If you cannot, make do with the outside.

Use a damp towel and Baking Soda to clean the headlight gently. Wash off with water. They become brighter for a very long time.

With this alone, you have saved yourself the cost of this book.

You can also do the same to anywhere you have chrome or alloy rims but not aluminium in your car because wet Baking Soda will react with it.

If you must use Baking Soda on them, use dry powder gently.

### 38. Stop Batteries Terminals Corrosion.

You can use Baking soda to neutralize the corrosion on battery terminals. You do not need a brush.

In any case, the salt will still appear after the brushing.

Disconnect the terminals

3parts of Baking Soda
1 part of water

Use to scrub the terminals' both on the battery and cables.

Fix back, then top with grease and enjoy.

### 39. Stubborn Carpet Stains

If you have stains on your carpet, be in the car or in the house, you can get them off with baking soda.

With vinegar, you get a WAO action.

Baking soda is a top odor absorber, its natural on materials plus the fact that it's cheap.

It goes down the carpet and uproots the stains.

Mix baking soda and distilled white vinegar, rub it into the stain. Leave overnight.

Clean the following day or use a vacuum cleaner if you have one.

### 40. Tape Residue Removal

Paste residue is difficult to remove from cars.

They could come from price tapes and even branding tapes.

Often you will need to scratch them to remove damaging the paintwork.

No need to scratch your car.

Get a damp towel, sprinkle some Baking Soda on it and use it to rub off the residue.

### 41. Car Leather Treatment

For your car seats, get a damp towel with Baking Soda and stroke on the leather gently, making sure it removes the stains.

This process will remove dirt as well from the surface. Top up with wiping up with a clean damp towel.

### 42. Sparkling Wheels and Rims

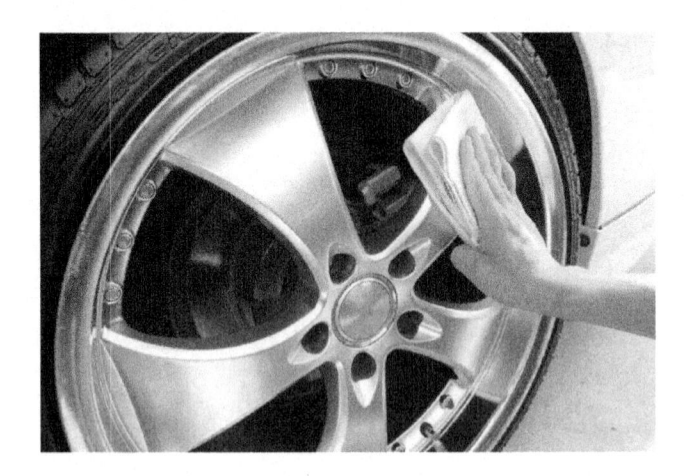

Make a thick paste of 3 cups of Baking soda and 1 cup of warm water.

Apply on rims and wheels and leave for a few minutes before scrubbing. For a Wao effect, add some drops of vinegar or Lemon juice.

### 43. Seat Belts Are Like New
Your seat belt has accumulated a lot of dirt, messing up your dress beside the grim it gives you.

Time to ask your friend Baking soda for help.

Use 50/50 paste of water and Baking soda to scrub the belt. Wipe with a clean cloth and you are free from seat-belt grime and stained shirts after driving.

### 44. Smokers Ashtray And Others.
OK, you still smoke in the car? Then, you must experience some foul odor in the car.

Kill the odor by cleaning the ashtray with baking soda. Apply the powder in the tray and leave for 5minutes. Wipe off with a damp cloth.

You can do this for holes for coffee and bottled water and minerals.

This is the cleaning, and it differs from stuffing the ashtray with Baking Soda as air freshener.

The thing is, Baking soda is unbelievably cheap, non-toxic, and effective. Its God gift to man

# 11. BAKING SODA IN FOOD

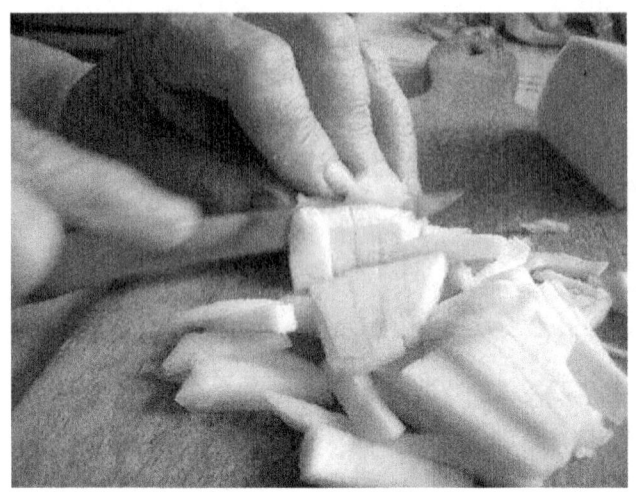

**45. Leavening Agent In Bakery.**

Bicarbonate of soda is used in bakeries as a Leavening agent. As we explained earlier, it produces carbon dioxide which makes the dough rise.

Individual baker has his or her recipe where they combine baking soda, baking powder, and other substances to make bread and cakes to taste.

We would rather leave this to individuals rather than give a recipe here.

Suffice to say that baking soda is universally used in bakeries. And this is probably its most popular usage.

**46. Make The Meat Soft And Tender**

Have you ever had to battle a piece of tough meat at a party?

On occasions, I have had awful luck and had to forgo meats because they were tough.

If the cooks of such hard meat had known baking soda, they would not have to give their guests such hard nuts to crack.

Right from when they were boiling the cow beef, they would have solved the problem by adding baking soda.

If you are unlucky to buy tough beef from the abattoir, you can save yourself some trouble and gas by incorporating Baking soda.

- Dissolve baking Soda in water
- 1 teaspoon of Baking soda in 1 liter of water
- soak the meat in the solution
- After 15 minutes, rinse and cook.

Alternatively, you can add some quantity of Baking Soda when you are steaming the beef. Don't overdo it so as not to spoil the meat.

The quantity to use depends on the size of the cow beef. It is better not to be enough than to overdo it.

### 47. Make Your Own Soda Water

Industrially, Baking Soda is a source of carbon dioxide in soda water making.

You can give yourself the luxury of making one in your home.
Put mall quantity of baking soda in a glass cup, add sugar to taste, squeeze some lemon to it and add water.

Mix thoroughly and drink. You have just taken soda water.

### 48. Neutralize Extract Brew

If you are an extract brewer, you fret little if your brew is acidic and you know this by testing the pH.

If this happens, adjust the pH by adding some powder of baking soda.

If for example, you have 10 liters of brew liquor, about 1 teaspoon of baking soda will neutralize the excess acid. Add gradually so as not to overdo it.

### 49. Softens Beans And Other Hard Cereals

Beans are hard to get softened and so are some other cereals like maize.

Sometimes, you will need a pressure cooker to soften them. Do not worry if you do not have one, Baking soda will help.

The high pH of the cooking solution will soften and tenderize the beans.

You dissolve one teaspoon into about 6 cups of water and cook.

If you want to do 'moin-moin', a delicacy in the southwest of Nigeria, you soak your beans as stated above before grinding. You get very soft silky beans.

### 50. Stop The Fruits From Going Yellowing

Sometimes you do not want your fruits going yellow quickly.

Soak fresh fruit in baking soda solution for a while to prevent yellowing.

# 12. GARDEN.

### 51. Cabbage Caterpillar Crusher

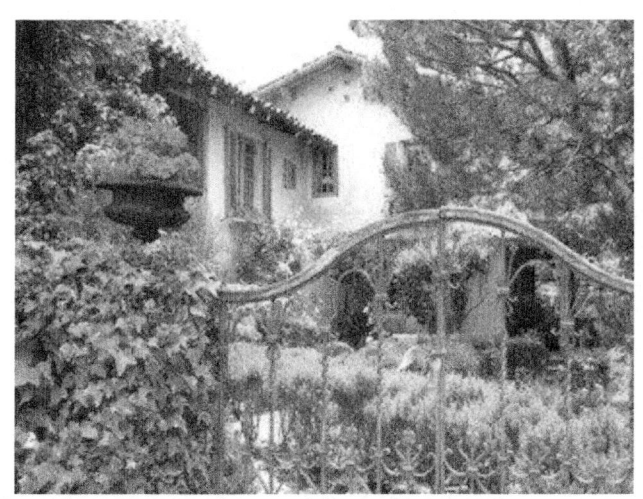

Cruciferous vegetables, cabbages, broccoli, or mustard plants are attacked by hungry caterpillars.

Mix 50/50 mixture of Baking Soda and in a shaker container or powder dispenser to dust your plants.

These plants are rugged and as Baking Soda is buffered with the white powder, it will not affect the plants.

The caterpillars will ingest the powder and will be killed by the baking soda.

Use for 3 or 4 days.

### 52. Fire Ants In Trouble

You have fire ants or the red ants disturbing you. Do not worry, the wonder powder, Baking Soda is a savior.

**Mix**
- ✓ 1 milk cup of Baking soda
- ✓ 1 milk cup of powdered(not granulated) sugar
- ✓ Put the mixture on a flat plastic near the ants.

They will drag the mixture to their place as the sugar will attract them.

They eat it. They enjoy the sugar but the Baking soda will kill them by disorganizing their body chemistry which culminates in their death.

They will also dry up with time.

### 53. Harmful Insect Infestations.

Sometimes the bugs and insects swam your garden with determination to do havoc.

If you experience this, face them with this solution.
- ✓ 5litres of water
- ✓ 1 tablespoon of Baking Soda
- ✓ A dozen drops of dishwashing liquid
- ✓ 1 tablespoon of olive oil
- ✓

Spray once daily for three days to eradicate them

Use a lighter formulation weekly to prevent re-infestation.

### 54. Kill Gnats In Compost Heaps

Compost heaps will smell no doubt and with time they have gnats.

4 teaspoons of baking soda in 5 litre of water and a teaspoon of biodegradable soap such as Castile soap will do the trick.

Spray or pour the mixture over the compost heap.

All gnats lurking around are dead.

### 55. Make Garden Furniture Shine

You can work on your garden furniture and make them new with baking soda.

You make a simple solution of half cup baking soda and a tablespoon of dishwashing soap in 5 liters of water.

Scrub gently with a scrubbing sponge, and rinse thoroughly with water.

For stubborn stains, make a paste from the above and scrub harder but don't use a hard brush so as not to spoil the surface.

We can use the same on the furniture inside the house.

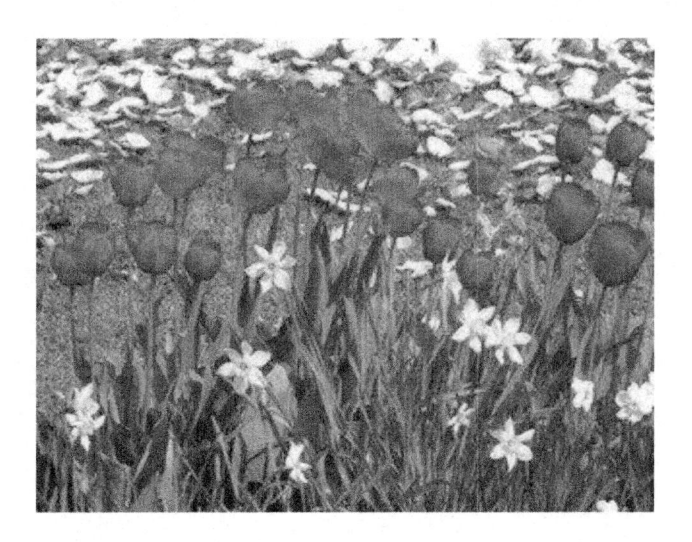

### 56. Plants Boost

Use this recipe monthly and watch your listless plants coming to life

Water with a combination of:
- ✓ 2teaspoon of baking soda
- ✓ 5 liters of pure, distilled or filtered water
- ✓ ½ teaspoon ammonia
- ✓ 1 teaspoon of Epsom salts.

### 57. Roses will thank you profusely.

This is Tough Organic Spray

The recipe below is effective for a wide variety of plant hassles including mildew, red spider termites, and even aphids.

- ✓ 5liters of water
- ✓ 4 drops of Superthrive, buy online)
- ✓ 1 tablespoon of baking soda
- ✓ 1 tablespoon of seaweed emulsion (organic fish fertilizer).
- ✓ 1 tablespoon of dishwashing liquid.
- ✓ 2 tablespoons of fine horticultural oil.
- ✓

Mix together, pour into a spraying pump and spray when you are ready to use.

Best results in the evenings. You can repeat monthly

### 58. Treat Tomato Diseases

Treat tomato fungi and other diseases with this recipe on weekly application

- ✓ 2 gallons of water

- ✓ 2 tablespoons of baking soda
- ✓ 2 tablespoons of aspirin.
- ✓

Mix into a spray and put it in a spray bottle. Shake properly before you spray.

### 59. Effective Pesticide.

There are many pesticides but some may be toxic to the soil. Fortunately, Baking Soda will act effectively as a pesticide while not poisoning the soil.

**Recipe.**
- ✓ 1 tablespoon of olive oil,
- ✓ 2 two tablespoons of baking soda
- ✓ A few drops of liquid soap in 5liters of water.

Put in a sprayer and spray gently to your garden twice a week to keep the bugs at bay.

### 60. Soil pH Meter.

I like this. Instead of buying testing Kits, you can use Baking soda to test whether your garden soil is acidic or alkaline.

**Ingredients.**
- ✓ 1 Two samples of the garden soil
- ✓ ½ cup Baking soda
- ✓ ½ cup Vinegar
- ✓ Water

**Process.**
Pour vinegar into one of the two soil samples. If it bubbles, then your soil pH is over 7 means the soil is alkaline.

If it doesn't, proceed to the second sample with Baking soda. Add it to the soil with ½ sup of water.

If it bubbles, your soil is acidic.

pH 1 to 7 Acidic
pH 7 Neutral (Water)
pH 7 to 14 Alkaline.

### 61. Bouquets Last A Little Longer.

Sometimes you bring some flowers from outside to the house.
If you do this, you have taken them from their natural habitat which means they won't last.

But you can make them live longer by sprinkling them with a water solution of our magic powder.

Go to Alkaline water.

# 13. HEALTH USES

### 62. Alkaline water, A Must Have.

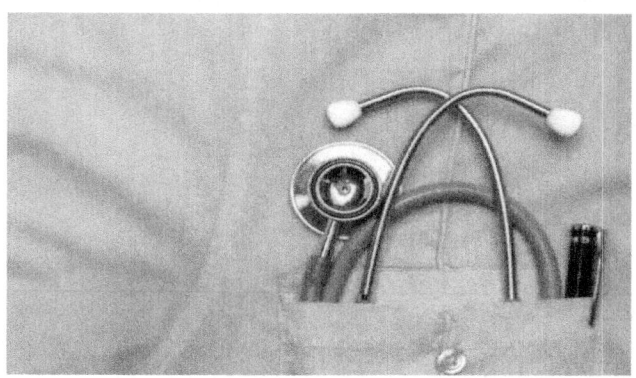

Baking soda alkaline solution is a magic solution that comes to your aid in many situations. You must and need to have it.

**How to make it.**
- ✓ Mix thoroughly.
- ✓ ½ tablespoon of Baking soda
- ✓ 5litres of water.
- ✓ Drink a little once a day or as your doctor prescribes.

Benefits Of Alkaline Water

Though no scientific backing yet, and like many unorthodox recipes, many have found an Alkaline solution of Baking soda very useful.

Alkaline water has ultra-hydrating properties as we discuss under sports

It boosts immunity.
It helps to maintain a healthy bone.

Act as antioxidants that help prevent cell growth which damages free radicals in the body and result in a quickening of the aging process.

The greatest benefit of alkaline water is that it reduces the acid level in your stomach

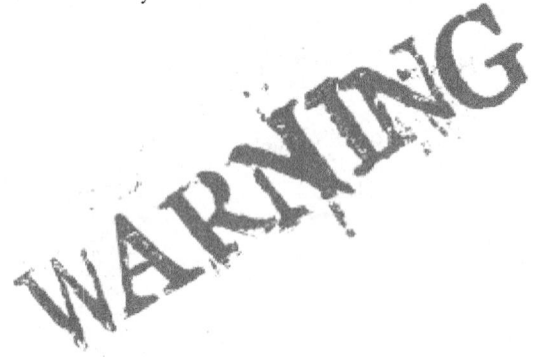

**WARNING**

Baking soda is not poisonous and is safe for consumption but its excess could be injurious.

First, it may over neutralize the acidity of the stomach which the enzymes need to work.

In addition, too much of it inside the body and on the skin may cause hassles in the alimentary canal and on the skin.

Moderation is the word.

### 63. As Digestive Aid

To digest heavy food quickly and to relieve flatulence, Baking soda is the aid you need.

1/4 teaspoon of baking soda
a glass of warm water
Mix and drink in a cup.

This mixture will zap acid in your stomach.

But remember, acid does not cause all indigestion.
If indigestion does not improve in days, please see your doctor.

It also helps with acid reflux and heartburn. It reacts with the acid in the stomach to produce sodium chloride which helps to relieve the burning.

## 64. Drop The Fats And Have A Flat Belly.

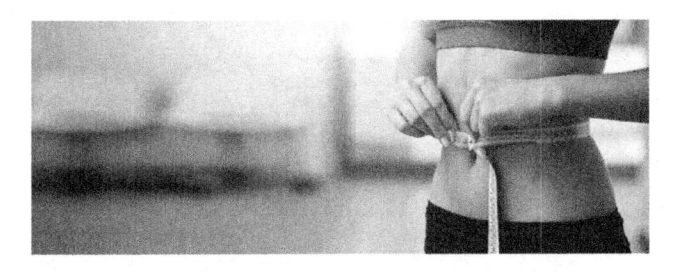

Baking soda can help you fight your obesity.

Apart from drinking alkaline solution on an empty stomach, the following recipes with other additives will help you drop the fats.

Lemon juice is full of antioxidants and a powerful fat-burning substance in its own right and can be mixed with baking soda to do the magic.

Add some lemon juice to the alkaline baking soda and drink.

- ✓ 1 teaspoon of baking soda
- ✓ ½ cup water
- ✓ Some lemon juice

**Preparation**

➤ Put the baking soda in the glass, mix until dissolved, add lemon, drink on an empty stomach in the morning to eat later. ***Another recipe with Fruits***
- ✓ 1 cup strawberry
- ✓ 1 spring of fresh mint leaves
- ✓ Juice of two lemons
- ✓ 2 cups of water
- ✓ ½ teaspoon Baking soda.

Put all in a mixer and blend properly.

Drink twice a day.

**Yet another**
- ✓ ½ teaspoon Baking Soda
- ✓ 2 tablespoon apple cider vinegar
- ✓ 1 cup of water
- ✓ Mix Baking soda and vinegar, put in a glass of water.
- ✓

Drink before breakfast

### 65. Fight Coughs and Colds

For quick relief for coughs, flu, and colds, mix one teaspoon of honey with 1 teaspoon of baking soda and a teaspoon of lemon juice.

Mix thoroughly until the Baking soda has dissolved then drink.

**The 3 Day Cold Baking Soda Course**

The following is from Arm and Hammer, makers of Baking Soda.

**1st Day. 6 doses of ½ teaspoon of Baking Soda in glass water every 2 hours.**

**2nd Day. 4doses as on the 1st day above every 2 hours.
3rd Day. 2 doses as on 1st day twice a day.**

Subsequent days, once in the morning until the flu disappears It will relieve you.

### 66. Fight Rosacea.
Baking soda is anti-inflammatory which makes it very useful to people who have skin issues that get triggered by inflammation.

An example is those suffering from rosacea, psoriasis, and acne. They get some relief when they use Baking Soda.

use a mixture of water, and baking soda to relieve blotches and bumps on the face.

See pimples.

### 67. Kidney Functions Better
Some people believe that drinking alkaline water from baking soda will help make the kidney function better.

The reason being that baking soda being alkaline will reduce the acidity in the system to make the work of the kidney easier.

The kidney is the filtering house for the body.

### 68. Natural Antacid And Acid Reflux
Baking soda is a neutralizing agent we know already.

When the stomach acid flows back to the esophagus, you have what we call acid reflux.

This irritates the esophagus and causes acid heartburn which comes as some burning feeling that occurs anywhere between the abdomen and the throat.

- ✓ 1 teaspoon of baking soda
- ✓ ¼ liter of water and drink. Not all at once.
- ✓

Bicarbonate of soda neutralizes the acid from the stomach and relieves you of the burning chest and many other stomach hassles.

### 69. Do Nasal Irrigation If You Can.

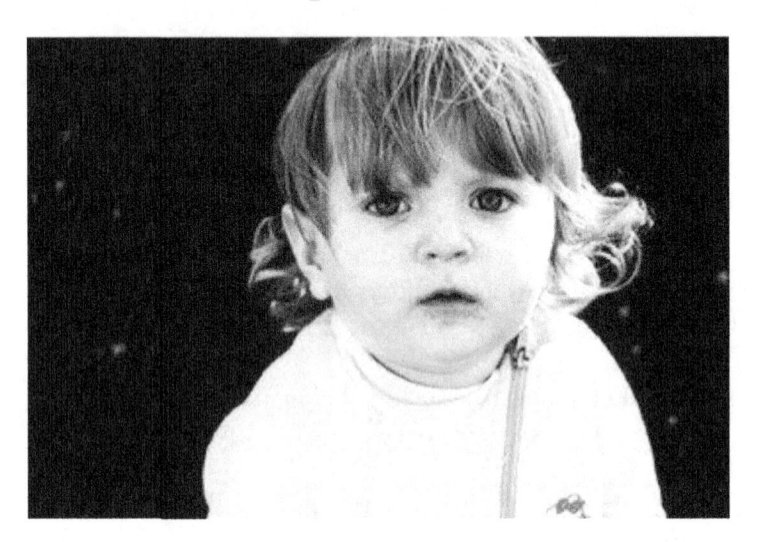

We also use baking soda as a buffering agent. If it's combined with table salt to create a solution for nasal irrigation.

This is done by addition of a teaspoon of sodium bicarbonate to cool water that was recently boiled,

Put a solution in a squeeze bottle. While keeping your mouth open, squeeze the bottle, to pour the water into your nostril.

Just drops.

Remember to breathe through your mouth, not your nose.

### 70. Clear Urinary Tract Infections(UTI)

For urinary tract infection (UTI) Baking soda and water solution act as a protective barrier.

This is due to Baking Soda's ability to reduce acid levels.

What an inexpensive remedy.

- ✓ 1/2 to 1 teaspoon of Baking Soda
- ✓ A glass of water;
- ✓ Mix and drink on an empty stomach.

### 71. Zaps Ulcer Pain

Simple. Ulcer is caused by too much acid in the stomach and baking soda neutralizes acid.

A bit of it will be a good first aid to ulcer before you see your doctor.

**These are common ulcer symptoms.**
- ➤ Stomach pain that wakes you up at night.
- ➤ Bloating, burning, or dull pain in your stomach.
- ➤ Discomfort when you eat or drink (gastric ulcer)
- ➤ Pains coming intermittently in days or weeks.
- ➤ Discomfort between meals or during the night (duodenal ulcer)Go drink alkaline water of Baking Soda

## 14. HOME USES.

### 72. Bathroom Cleaner.

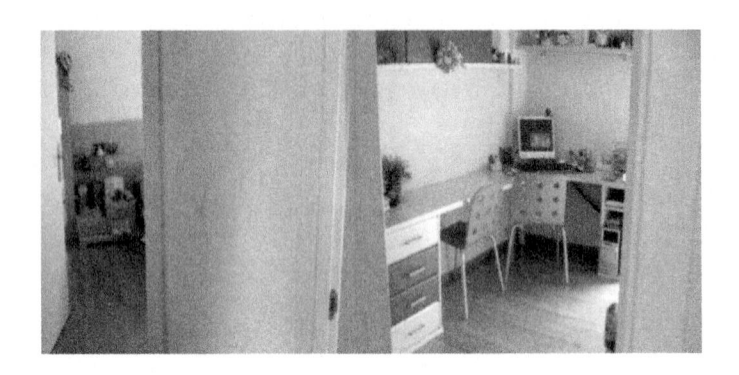

You can use baking soda to make a product to clean your bathrooms whether it's made of ceramic tiles or just cement.

**Recipe.**
- ✓  ¼ cup of baking soda
- ✓  2 tablespoons of dish detergent or liquid soap
- ✓  Add some vinegar

Mix until creamy or viscous.

You can now apply on the floor, leave for some time or overnight, for best results, then wash off with a sponge.

### 73. Bathroom Curtains Cleaner

Do you use curtains in your bathroom?

With time, the curtains will develop mildew.

Not to worry, make a paste of baking soda, smear on the curtain.

Leave overnight and wash the curtain normally to remove the mold.

Wash with an alkaline solution and some liquid soap.

See Alkaline solution.

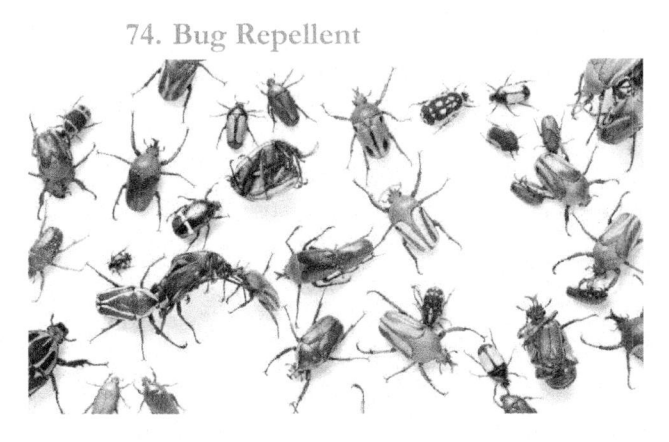

## 74. Bug Repellent

Some quantity of baking soda under sinks and along the basement of windows and dark corners can repel many insects and bugs.

If any of the insects as much as eat the powder, it will die a slow sure death.

And don't worry, if a junior tastes it, nothing will happen to him. If your pet eats too, no problem.

Baking soda is not toxic to man and pets.

### 75. Bees Or Insect Stings

Baking soda and water can help neutralize venom from bees and other insects. This will reduce the itching, pain, and swelling.

A paste of Baking Soda and water on the sting mark and later wash off with water.

It will relieve you.

### 76. Clean Brushes And Combs

You will need to first remove ant hair from the brushes and combs.

Soak them in a mixture of warm water and 1 teaspoon baking soda. They must be covered with the solution.

Leave for between 30 minutes and an hour. Rinse well in warm water. Clean and air dry.

### 77. Clean Your Tiles

Baking soda and vinegar can clean tiles on their own but when you mix both together, you get a bomb of a cleaner. When you mix both you get acid and a base. You mix ½ cup of baking soda, 1 tablespoon of vinegar, and 2tablespoons of liquid soap. Put on stains for a few minutes and wipe the stain off.

**Commercial**
- ✓ mix 1/2cup of borax,
- ✓ 1/2 cup of vinegar
- ✓ and 4litres of warm water
- ✓ ¼ cup of Baking soda.

Mix thoroughly and put into spaying bottles.

Spray on tiles, leave for some time, and wipe clean.

### 78. Cleaner In Dishwasher

Your pans and dishes carry some grease and baked-on food with time.

You will need to add some of the magic powder to your regular run in the dishwasher..

Baking soda reacts with the water to help remove grease and grime that build on your pans and dishes. See Alkaline water.

Being an alkaline substance, baking soda breaks the grease as in the saponification process in chemistry.

If you add vinegar, you have gotten good glasses cleaner. They come out shining.

### 79. Clear Your Drain

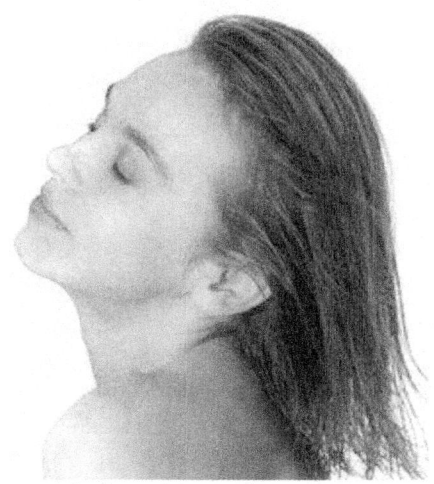

If your drain is blocked you may have to pieces it to clean out the blockage physically.

Not to worry, Baking Soda will come to your aid.
If you put in Baking soda on a weekly basis it will not block and you are lucky Baking soda is cheap..

**Recipe:**
- ✓ 1 cup of baking soda inside the drain
- ✓ Follow it with 1 cup of vinegar over.

The mixture will produce carbon dioxide that clears the drain If you want to up it, boil your vinegar before you add it to your baking soda.

### 80. Clears Grout Too.

You got some grouts on the floor? Don't worry our friend is here.

- ✓ Water 7cups
- ✓ Baking Soda ½ Cup
- ✓ Lemon Juice Or Liquid Ammonia 1/3 of a Cup
- ✓ Vinegar -1/4 Cup.
- ✓

Mix thoroughly and spray on grout, let it sink for 1 hour then scrub fiercely with a scrubbing brush.
It really works.

### 81. Cool Air Freshener For You.

You can make tons of money from this. It will be a hit with ladies if you get the packaging right.

You mix Baking Soda with essential oils. This could be one or a mixture of two or more to give you a distinct smell.

Examples of essential oils are Lavender, chamomile, Lavender, peppermint, eucalyptus, lemon, and rosemary.

**Recipe**
- ✓ Mix 15gm Baking Soda
- ✓ 5 to 6 drops of essential oil or a mixture.
- ✓

Mix thoroughly then put inside a sprayer (bottle) and top with distilled water (this is important) to taste.

You will decide the ratios until you get your perfect recipe.

Shake thoroughly and use it in a spray or bottle exotically to sell.

### 82. Recycling Bin Can Smell Nice/

Adding Baking Soda over the trash in the bin and damping the bottom and wall of the container with baking soda will eliminate smell and deodorize the bin.

### 83. Demolish The Ant Mound.

Ant mounds will dissolve with Baking soda.

Sprinkle it on the mound when damp and leave for 30 minutes.

Or 50/50 soda and water and put on the ant mound.

Follow up with a negligible amount of vinegar on the mound.

They will ingest the mixture which then reacts in their system and will send them to hell where they came from.

Use powdered sugar not granulated and mix thoroughly otherwise they will take the sugar and leave the bicarbonate of soda.

They eat they die

## 84. Experience Baking Soda Bath.

The first day I did Baking Soda bath, somebody commended me for the freshness oozing out of my body.

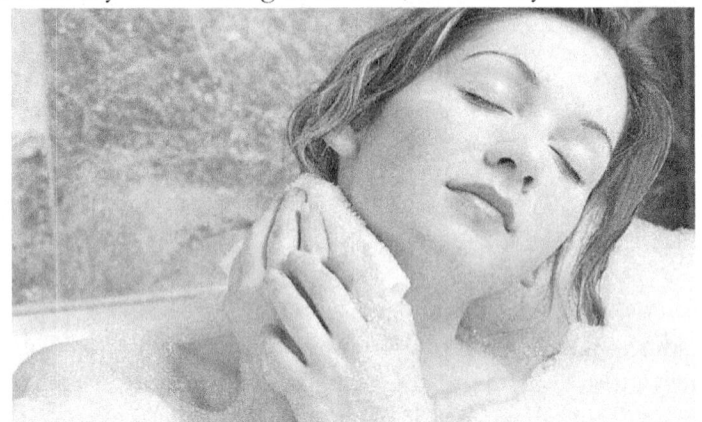

¼ to 2 cups of baking soda(depending on how much water )

A bucket of warm bathwater

Dissolve properly

Once completely dissolved, soak in the tub for up to 40 minutes.

If you are not using a tub, use the bucket, and have your baking soda birth with soap in your bathroom.

A pleasurable experience.

After the bath, dry your body and use a moisturizer.

## 85. Fruits Cleaner.

You have probably seen grocers using damp clothes to clean their veggies in the market. They need not do this when there is Baking soda.

It is faster and the fruits come out neater and fresher.

This is what they should do and which you can do too.

First, put water in a large bowl.(1 tablespoon to 2 cups of water?

Plus a teaspoon of baking soda.

Add the fruits or vegetables.
The water should cover them
Leave for a minute or two.
Use a brush to scrub.
Rinse off and use,

This will remove not only dirt but also pesticides from the farm

## 86. Fungicide.

Powdery Mildew is the commonest Fungi in the garden such as tomato blights.

It affects many veggies including but not limited to the following. artichoke, beans, beets, carrot, cucumber, eggplant, lettuce, melons, parsnips, peas, peppers, pumpkins, radishes, squash, matillo, tomatoes, turnips

Our baking soda does wonders here.
- ✓ 1 Full Tablespoon of Baking Soda (Sodium Bicarbonate)
- ✓ 1 Tablespoon of Horticultural Oil eg. Vegetable Oil
- ✓ ½ Teaspoon of Insecticidal Soap or liquid soap (Not detergent)
- ✓ 5litres of water

Mix thoroughly and spray, your Powdery Mildew will disappear.

### 87. Kill Crabgrass And Weeds In Your Lawn.

So you have a beautiful green lawn but you also have some crabgrass and weeds disturbing the lush.

First, wet the weeds with water.

Apply baking soda powder directly on the leaves of only the plants you want to kill.

Don't do it when there is wind as the powder may be blown to your grass.

Be careful, ensure you apply directly to the weeds you.

### 88. Laundry Bag.

You pack your dirty clothes in a basket or bag preparing for laundry but you are not ready yet.

The clothes now give you some awful odor. Just sprinkle a little Baking Soda on the clothes to eliminate the odor.

### 89. Laundry Whitener.

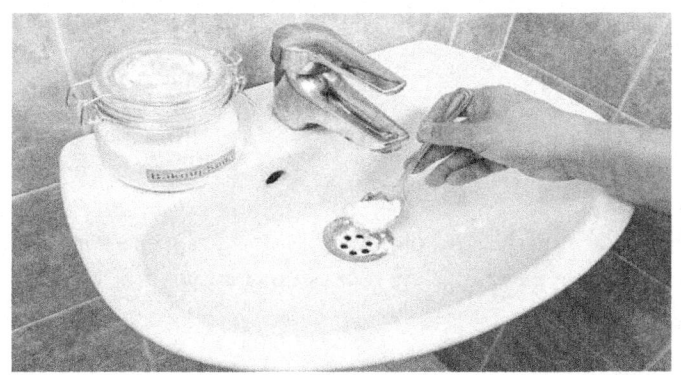

There are many things you can use to brighten your laundry beside the expensive stuff you buy in the supermarket.

Chlorine, dishwasher detergent, and hydrogen peroxide will brighten your clothes but magic Baking Soda will do the same at a much cheaper price.

Our friend, Baking soda freshens, whitens, and softens clothes.

**Recipe.**
- ✓ Baking Soda —1/2 Cup. Mix with your laundry soap
- ✓ For stains, make a paste of baking soda using water and apply directly to the stain on the fabric

**Commercialize.** Package the powder and put instructions at the back.

That is what big companies do.

### 90. Make Everything Sparkle.

You can use the 3 to 1 ratio paste to make all the chrome parts of the car to sparkle.

Take a damp towel and touch the wiper blades, windshields, license plates. Later rinse with plenty of water, and see them sparkle.

### 91. Old Books Are New.

Dirty and musty old books smell. Use baking soda to deodorize them.

Sprinkle on the cover and some pages. Put it in a paper bag and let it stay for days.

Remove the powder and expose the book to some sunlight. It may not remove the mildew marks but you will not have mildew marks again.

### 92. Pests Control

With sugar and baking soda, you should not have cockroaches or any insect disturbing you in your house.

And you know how dangerous roaches can be
Mix equal parts of sugar and Baking Soda,

Put in corners of the house or where the pests are. The sugar attracts the insects; they eat and the baking soda kills them. Clean them off the following day.

If you have them destroying plants in your garden. Dust the mixture around the plants. It will kill the crawlers.

Have you seen a man selling tiny insects killer? That is what he uses.

Let me give you this for free. It is not Baking Soda use though.

Soak two or three slices of bread in beer. Put them in a container with the rough outside to make it easy for roaches to climb.

A good harvest in the morning.

### 93. Plant And Flower Leaves

If you have plants in your compound or you have flowers. You can help them get more from their photosynthesis by cleaning the leaves.

Plants get their food through a biological process called photosynthesis where they use sunlight and carbon dioxide to manufacture their food.

Clean leaves will definitely do better than dirty ones.

About 1 teaspoon of our powder in 1litre of filtered undiluted water and use a hand towel to clean the leaves.

The flowers will thank you for this.

### 94. Insects Repellent

A mixture of baking soda and mustard oil will repel a variety of ants.
- ✓ 1 teaspoonful of baking soda
- ✓ 1/3 cup of mustard oil

Mix and store in a tightly cocked plastic bottle.

When you want to use it, decant into a spraying bottle and spray.

Two teaspoons of the mixture in a cup of warm water to spray where you don't want insects and bugs,

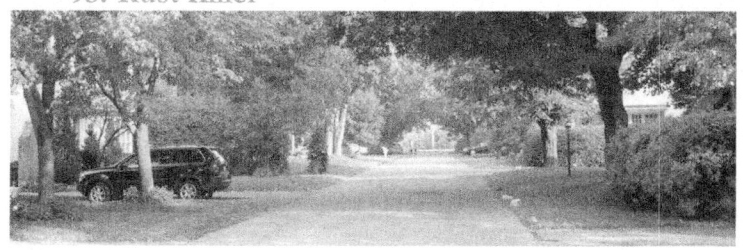

### 95. Rust Killer

To get rid of rust, make a paste of baking soda and water and apply on the rust and scrub off. Five minutes after, the rust is off. As simple as that.

### 96. Scouring Powder

Scouring powder is used to clean crusty covered surfaces on pots and pans, ceramic tiles, grill, baking trays, bathtubs, porcelain sinks, toilet bowls, and other bathroom fixtures.

**Recipe.**
- ✓ 2cups Baking Soda.
- ✓ 1.cup salt (not iodized)
- ✓ 1Cup washing soda.(sodium Carbonate)
- ✓ 10.drops lemon essential oil for a nice smell if you want.

Apply on the surface let the mixture soak in and scrub off.

### 97. Shine Shine Your Carpet

Many of the commercial carpet cleaners on the market today contain harsh chemicals that can be harmful to your children and pets.

Today's carpet cleaners could be made of harsh chemicals that may damage your carpets.

Baking soda will help clean them and make them free of the baby's urine odor besides removing dirt.

Sprinkle your carpet with baking soda, allow to sink for about 20 minutes, then vacuum.

**If there are stains use this recipe.**
- ✓ 1 cup of Baking soda
- ✓ 1 cup of Vinegar
- ✓ 1 cup of Water

Scrub the stains off.

### 98. Sparkle Floors

Cleaning your floors is one of the many baking Soda brilliant uses.

Let your floor be made of marble, porcelain, laminate, or tiles your friend Baking Soda is at hand to help.

Be gentle on furniture. Do not scratch them but scrub them gently.

**This is the recipe.**
- ¼ cup Baking soda
- ¼ cup White vinegar
- 5 liters Hot water

### 99. Silver Polish

To polish silver jewellery, make a paste of water and Baking Soda put it in the palm of your hand, and rub your silver between your hands.

For silverware and silver, rub the paste on with a soft cloth and rinse.

Have you ever seen a goldsmith rubbing some pieces of jewellery in a powder?

### 100. Stinky Sneakers

You will need to treat your plimsolls and sneakers and spank them up with a pleasant odor.

- one tablespoon of hot water
- one tablespoon of vinegar (white)
- one tablespoon of baking soda.

Mix to a paste, then use a brush to put the mixture onto the insole areas of your plimsolls.

Brush and clean.

### 101. Swimming Pool Alkalinity

We use baking soda in pools, spas, and garden ponds to raise the total alkalinity.

When the alkalinity is raised, the pH also goes up and makes pH maintenance easier.

When the pH is high, you do not use Baking soda to adjust because more addition will raise the pH the more.

Add the powder gradually to the pool while testing the pH. You may need a weak acid such as Formic acid to bring the pH down.

### 103. Toilets

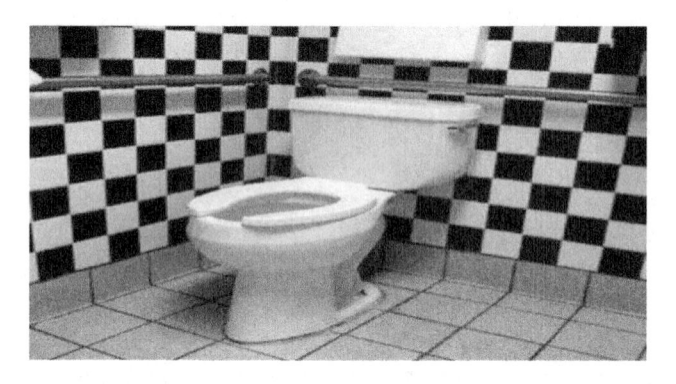

Treating your toilet with Baking Soda should be a weekly routine.

Sprinkle the toilet with a cup of baking soda.

Allow it to work for about 30 minutes then add vinegar to damp the power. Allow that to work with the powder for some minutes.

You can then scrub with a brush and flush the toilet.
Clean and odourless toilet for you.

### 104. Toothpaste

Many people hate fluoride which most toothpaste are made of.

Eliminate this by washing with a paste of Baking soda and water.

Your teeth are fresh and squeaky clean.

Not every day though.

Don't overdo so as not to damage your teeth. Use it now and then;

### 105. Towel Cleaner.

You can use our magic powder to freshen your towel which you use every day.

You get back the absorbency and bounce of the towel.
The smell and stinky aroma go away.

### 106. Wardrobes and Closets

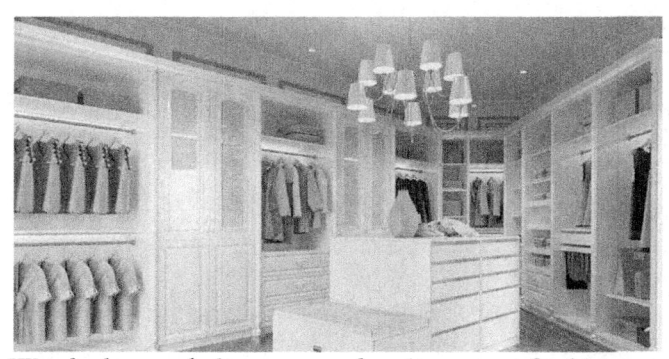

Wardrobes and closets may develop some funkiness.

Just place a box of baking soda on the shelve and enjoy fresh small.

### 107. Weed Your Sidewalk Weeds

Sidewalks, patios, crevices, and crack wall weeds can be dealt with using baking soda.

Sprinkle baking soda where weeds grow on and around the weeds.

Sweep powder into sidewalk cracks or spaces between pavers.

Reapply when needed.

The powder will destroy the foliage and may not kill the roots.

You may need to apply regularly especially during rainfall when rain has washed the powder away.

### 108. Window Cleaners

Proprietary window cleaner makers are cheats.

Put baking soda on a damp towel to clean your dirty windows and you get the sparkle.

See how to clean car windows.

### 109. Homemade Toothpaste

- ✓ 1 Tablespoon Baking Soda
- ✓ 2 Tablespoon Of Coconut Oil,
- ✓ 15 Drops Of Peppermint Essential Oil.

.

### 110. Computer Cleaning.

Believe me, you can use Baking Soda to clean the computer screen.

You ask, your phone's screen guard? and I say yes.

I use it for mine, both phones and the computer used to type this.

# 15. WITH KIDS

### 111. Baking Soda 'Clay'

You can make 'clay' from Baking soda for the little ones to play with during holidays and their spare time.

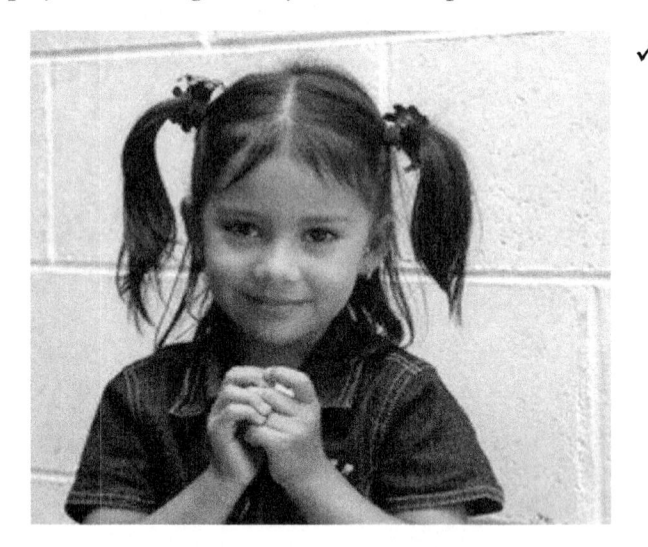

- ✓ Mix 2cups of baking soda, 1 cup of corn starch, and 1.25 cups of water.
- ✓ Boil to thicken,

You Have Your 'Clay' To Play With.

### 112. Bed Wetting Mattresses

Bed-wetting. We all have them wetting their beds now and then. You do not want to stay with the smell, do you?

Remove the bed-sheets to allow you to sprinkle the mattress with baking soda.

Leave for some minutes for it to soak up the urine and the odor. Expose to sunlight.

Add some Baking soda when washing the wet sheets.

### 113. Clear The Crayon Stains

Your restless six years old have messed up your wall with crayon thinking he is doing some great artwork.

You dislike these drawings all over the place, stairs, table, etc. It annoys.

Relax, just sprinkle some Baking Soda on a damp towel and rub off. Clean water to clean up.

Does it not occur to you that you can make this to a solution to sell to schools to clean their whiteboards?

I tell you some of them find it difficult cleaning the writings on the whiteboards.

I know because I own a school.

### 114. Dolls And Stuffed Animals Get A Bath.

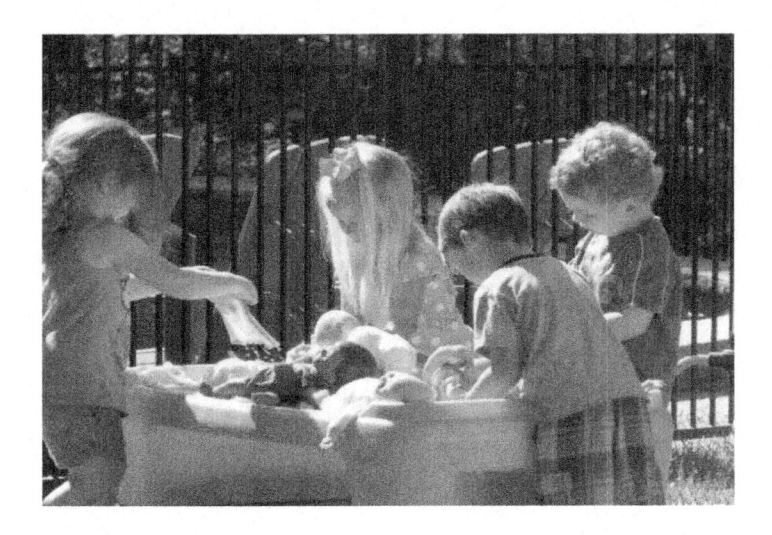

Yes, junior has stuffed animals and dolls. They play and sleep with them, then getting funky is not out of the way.

If they do, wash them and sprinkle a little baking soda on them. Give them a good shake or brush to remove the powder.

Dolls become cleaner and odorless.

### 115. Kids Lunch Boxes Smell Nice.

After several weeks of use, the junior's lunch box will generate some odor absorbed from the food packed inside.

Wash as hard as you could, the smell stays but Baking Soda will smash the odor and give you a refreshing smell.

Just put in some powder and scrub with a damp towel and wash off.

## 16. IN THE KITCHEN.

### 116. BBQ (Barbecue) Grill

Make a paste of baking soda, scrub on the grill, let it sink for 15 minutes and then wipe away. Then wash.

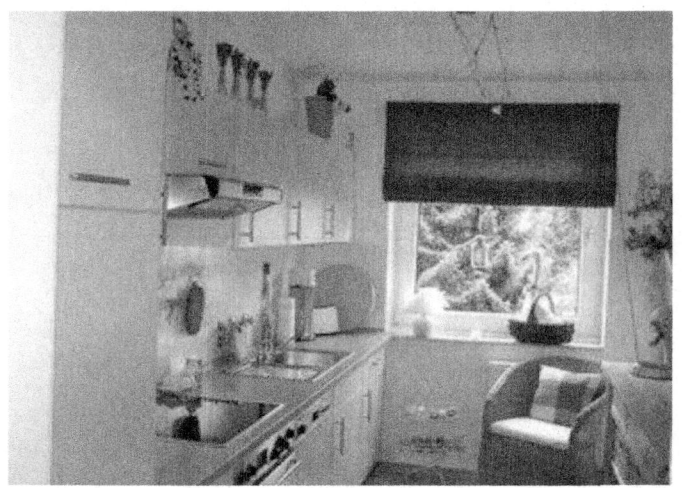

### 117. Delete Hand Odor

Have you just handled garlic, onion or ginger, if yes their small lingers and your friends may not like it.

Remove the small with a mixture of baking soda, detergent, and water.

### 118. Funky-Smelling Dishwasher

You can remove this smell from your dishwasher with baking soda.

Put 1 cup of baking soda at the bottom of the washer and run it on a rinse circle.

If you still perceive the small, put powder at the bottom and let it stay there a while.

93

Run the next load with it.

### 119. Garbage Disposals

You cannot beat your child and ask him not to cry.

If you dump leftovers in the garbage disposal bucket or drum, you must expect some foul odor.

Baking Soda will help you suppress the smell and keep the foul odor from filtering into the house.

Just sprinkle some baking soda on top of the garbage.

### 120. Iron Plate and Coffee Pot Rebirth

If your iron plate is crusty and dirty and it stains your coffee pot, our friend Baking Soda will help.

All you need to do is mix some quantity of baking soda in water to a paste and apply the paste directly on the stains and let it sink in for about 5 minutes.

Wipe clean with a damp towel.

You can always wash your coffee mugs in a solution of warm water and baking soda.

If stains are stubborn, soak mugs in a solution of baking soda overnight.

To ¼ teaspoon of baking soda, add some washing detergent and add water to make the solution.

These 3 ways you get sparklingly clean iron plates and coffee mugs.

### 121. Plastic Food Storage

You use plastic to store food like garri rice, beans and powder foods. You will need to remove the odor once in a while.

Use a hot solution of water and one teaspoon of Baking Soda with few drops of liquid dish detergent.

Let it stand overnight if necessary.

Wash and rinse.

### 122. Pop-Up The Omelette A Bit

Add half a teaspoon of baking soda to three eggs and make a pop-up omelet.

The omelet comes out bigger and tastier.

### 123. Make Your Own Fire Extinguisher

Now do not go face a big fire with this, but small fires in the kitchen can be dealt with using this recipe.

Remember, we said that Baking Soda produces carbon

dioxide rapidly and carbon dioxide extinguishes fire in a jiffy. That is the chemistry used by fire services.

**Recipe.**
- ✓ Get a jar and fill halfway with vinegar.
- ✓ Add 2 tablespoons full of Baking Soda.

Shake the jar immediately and point straight at the fire.
*Be careful, don't spill the mixture. Try to hold the bottle at an angle such that the carbon dioxide flows out onto the fire.*

If it is a grease fire in the frypan, quickly throw the powder at it. It will stifle it.

Can you think about how to use this recipe for car fire extinguisher?

### 124. Multipurpose Kitchen Cleaner

As we know already, Baking Soda does so many things in the house.

A simple Baking soda concoction can replace most of the proprietary cleaners you buy putting holes in your pocket.

This is a multipurpose cleaner made with Baking Soda that you can use to clean your kitchen and many other things.

Better still, you can package and sell.

**Recipe: Mix**
- ✓ 1 tablespoon baking soda
- ✓ 1 tablespoon borax
- ✓ 1/4 tablespoon liquid dish soap
- ✓ 2 tablespoons vinegar or lemon juice
- ✓ 2 cups hot water

Mix thoroughly and store in a bottle.

When you want to use it, put in a spray bottle and spray. Leave for a period and wipe off.

When mixing this stuff, please use a glove. Borax is a strong base and may burn the hands.

### 125. Neutralize Fridge Odors

You can make neutralizers for fridge odor using Baking Soda.

**Recipe:**
**Mix:**
4tablespoon of Baking Soda

1litter of water.

Use the resultant solution to scrub the inside of the freezer and leave the door open for a day or two to allow the moisture to dry completely
Your freezer is free of odor.

You can package the solution and sell as a fridge and freezer cleaner.

### 126. Odor-Free Microwaves

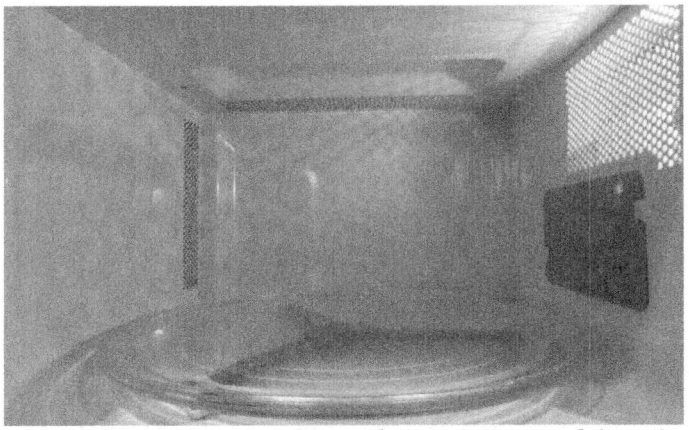

Sometimes, some repelling odor comes out of the microwave, and with time they build up.

To beat the odor, gently scour the floor with the paste or just sprinkle with Baking Soda and leave for a couple of hours. Rinse and dry.

Please disconnect from the mains while cleaning the microwave or when cleaning any appliance using electricity,

### 127. Scorched Pot Cleaner

You have burnt food in a pot before rendering the pot scorched.
Baking Soda will make them cleaner and sparkle.

Put baking soda in the pan or pot as if you want to fry or cook the powder; Add enough water to cover the scorched area. Add some vinegar.

The solution should be viscous. Put the solution to boil. Clean off but if some stains remain, add some viscous solution and brush off.

### 128. Sparkle Pots And Pans

Have you ever noticed some people cleaning dirty pots at bus stops and then sell the powder to them?

That powder is Baking Soda.

You can use Baking Soda solution to clean your pots and pans.

Soak them in the solution before washing to clean them without scratching.

You can scrub with Baking Soda.

This also works well with enamel, porcelain, and ceramic.

### 129. Stale Smell From Used Containers

Wash them with hot Baking Soda solution to kill the smell. If the smell is powerful, you can soak the containers in the

Baking Soda solution overnight.
Wash and rinse. Smell goes.

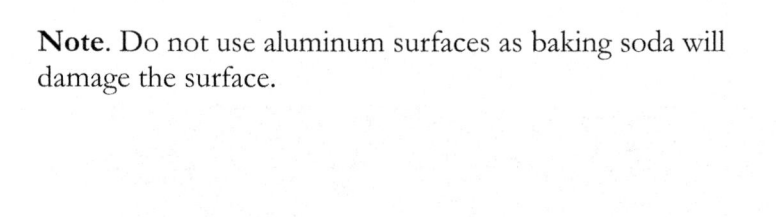

**Note.** Do not use aluminum surfaces as baking soda will damage the surface.

### 130. Sweetening Tomato Fruits.

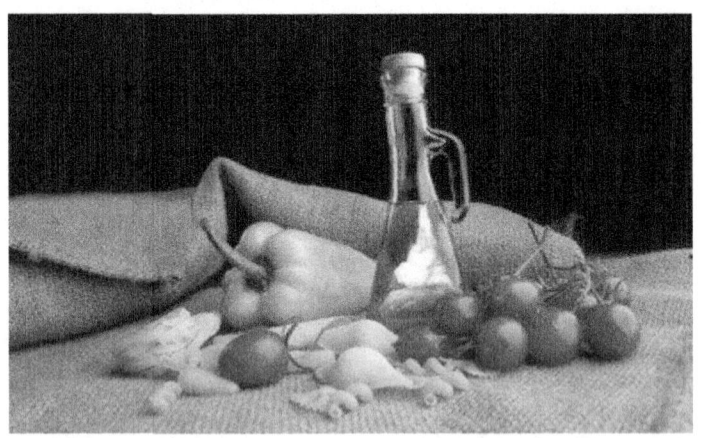

If you plant tomatoes, you can sweeten it more by adding Baking soda. It will give you a better taste than the ones you buy in the grocery.

Sprinkle a negligible quantity of baking soda, like 1/8 of a cup near the plant, making sure the powder does not touch the plant itself.

Alternatively, you can dissolve a tablespoon of baking soda in 5litres of water, add 2.5 tablespoons of vegetable oil, and half teaspoon of liquid soap. Mix and put in a spray bottle to spray the plants.

You can also add a negligible quantity of baking soda to sweeten canned tomatoes without risking high calories when you use sugar.

### 131. Thermoses And Flasks Too.

Flasks and dirty thermoses will clean better when you soak them in hot water and about 3tea teaspoon of baking soda overnight.

### 132. Wash The Blender

Fill up the blender to half, add 1 teaspoon of baking soda, and a little detergent. Blend and rinse.

# 17. PERSONAL HYGIENE

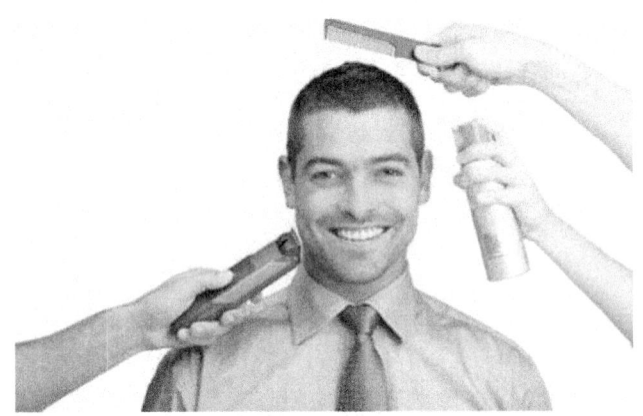

### 133. Deodorize Your Shoes

Smelling feet and shoes can embarrass, especially if you remove your shoes in the public.

A stinking shoe will make people around to close their nostrils while you get embarrassing glances.

This need not happen to you.

You can put such shoes in a bag and freeze it for a day in your freezer or use our friend baking soda.

Put 2 tablespoons in a clean cloth and push it to the front of each shoe overnight. Remove the clothes when you want to wear shoes.

Alternatively, sprinkle baking soda inside the shoes.

**Commercialize**. Sell Baking Soda and put the instruction at the back.

### 134. Fight off Athlete Foot.

During the rainy season, especially, some people experience itching between the toes.

The space between the affected toes becomes very white and wet. This is a fungi infection which is no match for Baking soda.

Mix Baking soda and lime and apply between the toes overnight and watch the fungi vamoose the next day.

**Or mix**
- ✓ 1/2 cup of baking soda
- ✓ 3 liters of warm water.

Soak feet for 20 minutes, morning and evening
After dry feet but do not wash. Let the solution soak in to do its job.

**Or**

Make a paste of baking soda and apply it. Allow to sink for some minutes and wash off.

### 135. Make A Deodorant

To use Baking soda as a deodorant, you need some additives like virgin coconut oil, Shea butter, lavender, or a fine smelling perfume.

**Recipe:**
- ✓ 3parts Baking soda
- ✓ 2parts Shea butter
- ✓ 3pars virgin coconut oil
- ✓ 2 parts cornstarch
- ✓ 6 drops essential oil (lavender) or to taste if 6drops not enough

**Processing.**
- Get a double boiler. You do this by getting a smaller container in a big one. Put water in the big one and heat it up gradually.
- Let the water cool. Now put shea butter and coconut oil in the smaller container and let them melt. Turn the heat off, add cornstarch and baking soda and stir until smooth. Mix the essential oil such as lavender and allow to cool,
- Scrape into the size of your choice and put under the armpit where it melts and soaks in.

Load into an antiperspirant tube and sell.

### 136. Mouthwash Kills Mouth Odour

Have you noticed some people ooze out nauseating odor when they speak? Some of them don't even know because nobody wants to tell them so as not to offend them.

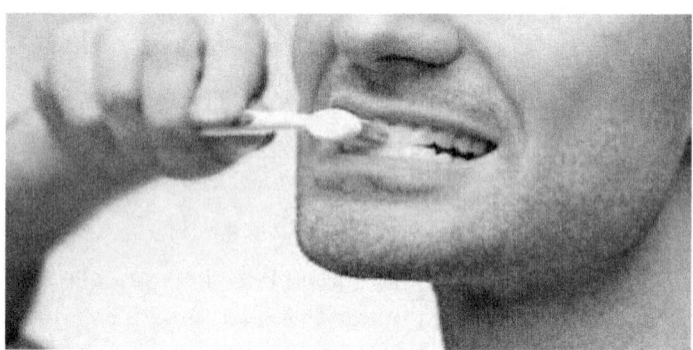

If you have such a person around you, Baking soda is your friend, it will help.

Remember, we said Baking Soda kills bacteria and fungi, we will put the property to use here.

**Recipe.**

- ✓ Half a teaspoon of Baking Soda
- ✓ Half a glass of warm water,

Mix and put in mouth and swirl for some time and spit out.
**Note:** *that this does not replace good mouth hygiene.*
Load into a well-packaged bottle and sell.

### 137. Sparkling Flatware

3 parts baking soda, 1 part water.

Rob on the flatware (eating utensils; cutlery, such as forks, knives, and spoons) with a sponge

Rinse thoroughly with water and dry.

Alternatively, wash them in alkaline water prepared from baking soda.

They come out sparkling.

### 138. Splinter Is Out.

Did you get a splinter in your body?

Dissolve some bicarbonate soda in some water and soak the spot twice a day.

Or

Make a paste of the powder and water and put on the surface and wait for several minutes for the splinter to come out.

Without pain, the splinter will come off in a few days

You have been using a toothbrush for some time and you think it is free of bacteria. Not completely.

¼ cup of our powder in ¼ cup of water.

Mix and soak the brush and other things used in the bathroom to kill off any bacteria.

Make a larger solution if you have more things in the bath. It does not cost much, baking soda is damn cheap.

## 18. IN SPORTS

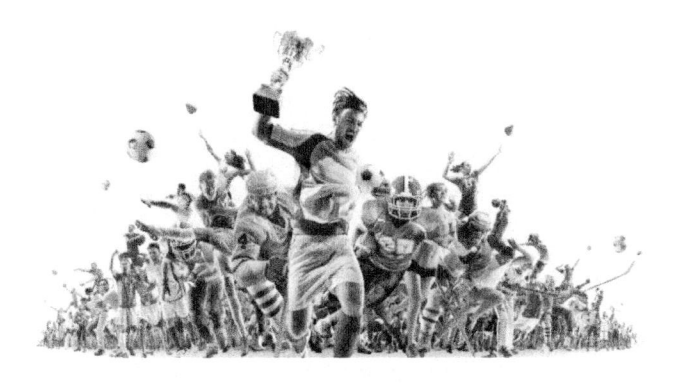

### 139. Cleaner Sports Equipment

Soccer boots can be smelly and so are other sports shoes and equipment.

Use 4tablespoon of baking soda to 1 liter of water to clean the equipment. Alternatively, get it to a paste and use it to scrub them.

Either way, the grim and smell are off.

### 140. Electrolyte Booster, Sports Drink

You need a booster to keep you hydrated and keep the right level of body electrolytes necessary for a run.

You need a drink of Baking Soda, and honey which is cheaper than sports drinks.

**Recipe.**
- ✓ coconut water-1cup
- ✓ lemon juice-3drops
- ✓ ½ teaspoon of honey
- ✓ Pinch of salt

Put it in a bottle, use it as you jog.

## 19. MORE USES.

### 141. Hot Water Burn

If you are unlucky to have hot water splashed on your hand, Baking soda will soothe it and reduce the pain.

Make a paste of 50/50 water and Baking soda and paste on the burn and allow the paste to work on the burn for about 10 minutes.

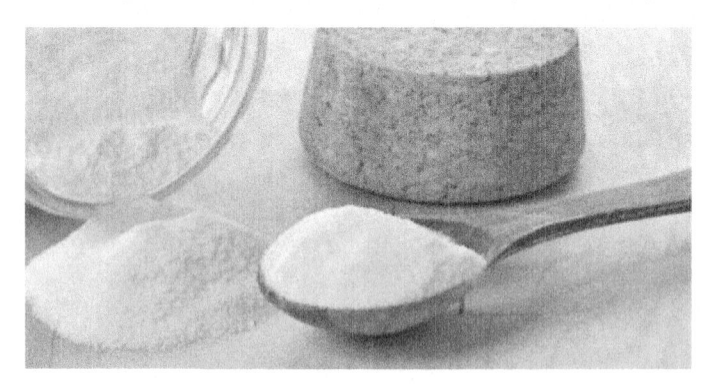

Wash off. The pain will go, and the burn will heal in time.

### 142. Peel Your Eggs With Ease

You do not have to struggle to remove your boiled eggs shell. Have you ever had to struggle to remove the shells?

I have had the luck a couple of times

Just half a teaspoon in the water to boil the eggs and you have a trouble free shell removal.

### 143. A Volcano To Thrill The Kids.

With Baking soda and some of its friends you can thrill the kids by making a Volcano.

The sound that comes out of it is exciting.

**Ingredients.**
- ✓ dish soap-5mils
- ✓ water-50mls
- ✓ white vinegar 200mils
- ✓ Drops of food colouring.
- ✓ Baking soda
- ✓ 1 liter soda bottle

**Experiment.**
- ➢ Fill a cup halfway with Baking Soda and top up with water. Mix thoroughly until it dissolves.
- ➢ In the empty soda water bottle put the rest—white vinegar, washing liquid, water and one or two drops of colouring agent.

**The Eruption.**
Pour the Baking Soda solution to the soda bottle containing the others and step back quickly.

The reaction of the chemicals, especially vinegar and Baking Soda produces carbon dioxide which causes the explosion in an attempt to escape.

Have you seen a beer bottle exploding before when you shake it. It is the same principle..

This is the chemistry behind using baking soda and vinegar to clean your drains.

WARNING: Please don't try this inside the house. It should be done outside asking your spectators to stay afar.

### 144. Reduce Food sour Taste

If a sauce or drink is too sour because of too much acid you can neutralize it with a small quantity of Baking soda. Just a pinch.

Similarly, if there is too much lemon in tea make it drinkable with a negligible quantity of Baking soda

### 145. Forget ToothAche

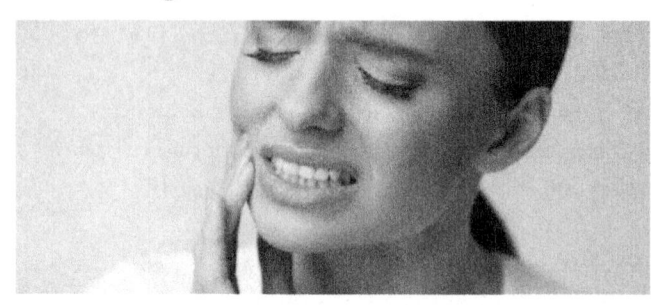

Baking soda is alkaline and therefore an acid Neutralizer. Bacteria are responsible for the pains in the teeth and they thrive in acid conditions.

Naturally, if you apply Baking Soda around the teeth, the bacteria will go and so also the pain.

Mix a negligible amount of baking soda, warm water and your regular toothpaste.

Apply on the affected area, leave to sink for about 10 minutes. Wash off thoroughly with clean water. The pain will go.

### 146. Baby Post Eating Fresh-Up

Wipe baby's face with a moist washcloth after feeding. You can extend this to his hands and clothes.

Baby smells fresh, devoid of baby food.

### 147. Wash Your Private Part {PP}
Can you use Baking Soda to wash your private part? Absolutely yes.

**Recipe:**
- ✓ Baking Soda 4teaspoons
- ✓ Water (bath water that is warm not hot.
- ✓

Your itching in the vulva will cease.

A more potent solution used directly will quicken the result. Men can use it to deal with rashes in their private parts.

### 148. Test For Baby Sex
There is a home test to predict the gender of an unborn baby. This has no scientific backing but many people still use it to guess the sex of their baby.

You combine the woman's urine and Baking soda and see if it fizzles.

**Procedure:**
- ✓ Collect the woman's urine first thing in the morning.
- ✓ Pour on Baking Soda and see whether it fizzles or not.

If it fizzles, the woman is carrying a baby boy, but if it stays the same, the woman is carrying a baby girl.

### 149. Garden Decorations to Enjoy

Garden decorations will enjoy Baking Soda just as those inside the house do.

Sprinkle on any surface you want to clean and wipe off with a damp cloth.

No harm, they get cleaned.

Your pets are safe also because Baking Soda though effective, is non-toxic.

### 150. Treat Cutting Boards

Cleaning cutting boards prevent contamination. Do this by sprinkling the powder and vinegar on the surface of the board.
Leave to sink, then rinse.

If you own a grinding stone in your kitchen, use the same recipe to clean it.

### 151. Wall Hole got filled up

Make a thick paste of baking soda and toothpaste use it to fill small holes on the plastered wall.

Smoothen and allow to dry.

### 152. Mobile Air Freshener For You

You can make your own air freshener cheap at home instead of the expensive ones out there with all their toxic chemicals.

Our friend Baking soda, water and some drops of essential oil are all you need. And a spraying Bottle.

Get a tablespoon of Baking soda, add some drops of essential oil, mix them together and put in the spraying bottle.
Top with water. It's ready for use. It diffuses any awful odor around you.

You can go out with it and use it whenever you perceive a foul odor.

**Use also in the car and offices.**

### 153. Sports Equipment Remembered

Soccer boots, golf bags in the gym, boxing gloves, canvases, spikes shoes, all smell better when you sprinkle our friend Baking soda on them.

### 154. Kills Sweet Craving

Some people crave for sweets but would not want to eat sweets. Baking soda can help kill the craving.

Some warm water and a tablespoon of Baking soda is all you need. Just rinse your mouth with the solution. Spit out the mixture.

Cravings should go.

### 155. Balloon Blow Blow

We can blow up a balloon to thrill the kids just as we tried to do the volcano. (see Volcano)

Get a balloon and inflate fully to the limit. This will open up the inside for what to follow.

Now, put 2 tablespoons of Baking soda using a small spoon or funnel.

Get an empty plastic bottle and put about 4 tablespoons of Vinegar.

Magic time. Try to get the balloon over the bottle, tilt the balloon in a way to make the baking soda enter the bottle as if you want to use the balloon to cover the bottle.

What do you see? The balloon inflates.

The carbon dioxide produced by the reaction rises to fill the balloon.

### 156. Gutter Cleaner Is Here

You have just cleaned your gutter and you want to brighten it up? Baking soda will help.

- ✓ It is non-toxic and can scrub the gutter and get a delightful smell to the bargain.

### 157. Glowing Skin Is Your Right.

To have a glowing skin you need to eat well, have 8 hours sleep, and maintain an impeccable skincare routine.

The question is, how many of us do that?

Many of us go for expensive proprietary products that burn our pockets with possible after use effects.

Our friend Baking Soda comes to our rescue. With orange juice, it gives you a blend of a natural product that is gentle on your skin while giving a glowing effect.

Orange has vitamin C that adds a glow to your skin naturally while Baking Soda exfoliates removing layers of dead cells.

**Recipe. Mix**
- ✓ 1 tablespoon of baking soda
- ✓ 2 tablespoons of orange juice.
- ✓

Wash your face and neck and then apply the paste evenly on your face and neck and leave for 15minutes.

Wipe off with a damp cloth and wash with plenty of water. You can apply this paste all over your body if you want it that way.

Do this once or twice a week to get a glowing face or body to the admiration of your peers.

# 20 CLEVER USES YOU CAN COMMERCIALIZE RIGHT AWAY

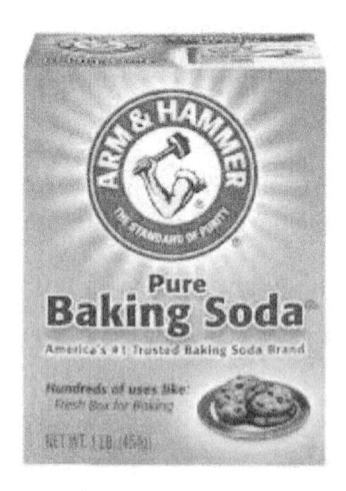

**Breaking bulk.**
1. Sell in bags
2. Sell in 1kg packs
3. Packaged in about 300gm for baking materials seller
4. Packaged in boxes as in Amazon or Konga
5. Pest repellent/pest killer
6. Anthill Destroyer
7. Scouring Powder
8. Car wash
9. Headlight Cleaner
10. Car fire extinguisher
11. Silver jewelery cleaner
12. Fragrance
13. Tiles cleaner
14. Toilet cleaner
15. Cloth whitener
16. Teeth whitener
17. Mouth odour killer

18. Nail paint remover
19. Lip softener
20. House window cleaner
21. White board cleaner
22. Toilet cleaner
23. Kitchen cleaner
24. Scorched pots cleaner
25. Eczema cure
26. Alkaline water
27. Furniture cleaner
28. Ants killer
29. Stretch mark removal
30. Dandruff fighter
31. Pimples
32. Dog dry bath to vets.

Dog owners have money. You can sell 250gm to them for 1000N if properly packaged,

33. Dogs Kennel Cleaner
34. Kennel Disinfectant
35. Fragrance In Kennel.

You can sell the same material for different uses using different packaging.

That is the trick. Most dog owners are not poor and rich people are dumb when they are buying things like this.

Trust me.

# 21. FAQS ON BAKING SODA.

Q. Are Baking soda and sodium Bicarbonate the same?
A. Yes, they are.

Q. What is the difference between Baking soda and Baking powder?
A. They are different. I answer the question in the earlier part of this book. Baking powder is baking soda and some acids.

Q. Any side effect of baking soda if consumed?
A. Too much of anything is bad, and we gave a caution earlier in this book. If you consume Baking soda in excess, you could have bloating and stomach upset.

Q what is the work of baking soda in baking?
A. It serves as a leavener.

Q. Is Baking soda toxic?
A. No, it is not. Your pets are safe if they ingest negligible quantity.

Q. Is Baking soda Corrosive on the skin?
A. No, it is not.

Q. Can one use Baking Soda alone to brush teeth?
A. Yes you can but not always otherwise you remove the natural protection on the teeth. Don't use it with Vinegar to brush your teeth. The mixture will be too abrasive.

Q. What do they call Baking Soda in the UK?
**A. Sodium Bicarbonate.**

Q. Are Baking Soda and Washing soda the same?
A. No, they are not. Baking Soda is Sodium Bicarbonate while Washing Soda is Sodium Carbonate. They sound

familiar and they are both good at washing. But Sodium Carbonate is more caustic and more expensive.

## 22. WRITE A REVIEW.

To share your experiences, you might choose to write a book review.

In fact, we kindly ask that you write an objective review of the copy of *The Instant Cure* that you have.

Whether or not you found the books informative, others will value your opinion on them.

Providing an unbiased review of a book can help readers determine whether books are appropriate for them.

Please take the time to go to the book's page on Amazon and write a few paragraphs about your thoughts on it.

Scroll down to customers reviews on the left and click the "write a customer review button"

I appreciate you doing this.

# 23. .OTHER BOOKS BY THE AUTHOR.

**The Instant Cure** (The Hidden Secrets To Healing Practically All Diseases) https://www.amazon.com/Instant-Cure-Secrets-Practically-Diseases-ebook/dp/B0BZ8SMTFJ/ref=sr_1_1?crid=194MN9YMZCUW3&keywords=the+instant+cure&qid=1679883447&s=books&sprefix=the+instant+cure%2Cstripbooks%2C228&sr=1-1

**Be Your Own Doctor With Apple Cider Vinegar** (125+ Unknown Health Uses Of Apple Cider Vinegar (ACV) That Save You Stress And Hospital Bills: Hypertension, Diabetes, Prostate, Weight Loss, Asthma) https://www.amazon.com/Your-Doctor-Apple-Cider-Vinegar-ebook/dp/B08QW5PFH8

# 20 ABOUT THE AUTHOR.

Jane Richard is an author, researcher, practitioner, and promoter of complementary and alternative medicine.

He is the author of numerous publications, including "The Instant Cure" and two others in the health, fitness, and diet niches.

With the side effects of orthodox medicine, he thinks that providing health care need not be as expensive as it is.

He believes we should rely more on nature as opposed to expensive medications and other substances used in our homes and surroundings.

Printed in Great Britain
by Amazon